Praise for *Healing*

"*Healing with Essential Oils* is not only a science but an art. Jodi Sternoff Cohen masters both beautifully in her expertly written book which deserves a revered place on your personal go-to book list for overall health and well-being."

Ann Louise Gittleman, PhD, CNS, Award winning *New York Times* bestselling author of over thirty books

"Jodi has done it! She has made the massive topic of essential oils into something we can understand and implement immediately! There is also a memory trauma technique she explains that is worth way more than the price for her book!"

Dr. Jay Davidson, DC, PScD

"In *Healing with Essential Oils*, Jodi Cohen does a masterful job of illuminating the world of these therapeutic oils. In an easy to understand and engaging manner, Jodi weaves together the history of healing with oils and the importance they can play in health. Jodi's book is a must-have for anyone interested in learning more about essential oils and how to include them into their own healing curriculum—practitioners and patients alike."

Andrea Nakayama, Functional Medicine Nutritionist, Founder, Replenish PDX and Holistic Nutrition Lab

"After thirty-five years in practice, if I had to pick just one tool to help people shift, it would be the use of essential oils. In her book, Healing with Essential Oils, Jodi presents a compelling case for the use of essential oils in an integrative healthcare practice. She presents credible scientific research and cuts through the widespread misinformation about essential oils in a simple, user friendly way. I have used her Vibrant Blue Oil Blends for years and have not been disappointed. Whether your goal is to manage surface symptoms, help cure underlying imbalances or facilitate healing of deeper root causes, the information presented here can be useful on all levels. I would highly recommend this book as a resource for anyone on a health quest or personal growth journey."

Peter J. Pinto, DC

Jodi has done a fantastic job putting together information that anyone can understand and use. Lots of great tools and of course her oils are the highest of quality! Thank you, Jodi!

Keesha Ewers, PhD, ARNP and bestselling author of Solving the AutoImmune Puzzle

"I have worked with essential oils in my nutrition practice for many years, yet learned so much from Jodi's excellent book. I love the paradigm of using high quality Vibrant Blue oils to address all five levels of healing. Jodi teaches us how essential oils open up the healing potential through the 'back door'. Essential oils are an effective adjunctive therapy for everyone on the road to wellness and this book is a brilliant training tool in their use. Thank you, Jodi!"

Anne Fischer Silva, RWS, NTP

"Jodi's personal story about healing with essential oils is inspiring. She combines deep intuition and research into the science of how essential oils work. Her consideration of EOs' effect on the endocrine system is fascinating. Though I've been working with essential oils for years, it's sometimes easy to forget just how powerful they can be. After reading this book, I find I'm inspired to help myself shift into parasympathetic mode (rest and digest mode) with essentials oils before I eat and as part of my evening routine."

Brodie Welch, L.Ac., M.S.O.M.

"I understand essential oils so much better after reading this book. As a Nutritional Therapist, I am always looking for natural ways to encourage healing. I recommend this book to all my clients who are interested in the power of essential oils!"

Beth Schultz, Real Food Inspired Me

"*Healing With Essential Oils* presents a revolutionary way to use oils to complement holistic medicine. It was so fascinating to read about different blends to stimulate lymph drainage or support all the organs involved in blood sugar regulation. The theory is very easy to apply because the book includes specific instructions on how to use each blend—for example using a blend of clove and lime behind the ears to calm the nervous system. I'd recommend this book to anyone looking for a straightforward guide on how to incorporate essential oils into their health protocols."

Erin Knight, FDN-P

Healing with Essential Oils

Healing with Essential Oils

How to Use Them to Enhance Sleep, Digestion and
Detoxification while Reducing Stress and Inflammation

Jodi Sternoff Cohen, NTP

Vibrant Blue Oils
Seattle, WA
www.vibrantblueoils.com

HEALING WITH ESSENTIAL OILS
Copyright © 2017 by Jodi Sternoff Cohen, NTP.

First Printing: 2017
Published by Vibrant Blue Oils, www.vibrantblueoils.com
Distributed by Chelsea Green Publishing
Edited by Donna Mosher, Segue Communications, Inc.
Interior Design by JETLAUNCH, www.jetlaunch.net

ORDERING INFORMATION
Special discounts are available on quantity purchases by corporations, associations, educators and others. For details contact the publisher at info@vibrantblueoils.com.

BOOKING, PRESS & SPEAKING ENGAGEMENTS
www.vibrantblueoils.com/press

The author of this book does not dispense medical advice or prescribe the use of any technique as a form of treatment for physical, emotional, or medical problems without the advice of a physician, either directly, or indirectly. The intent of the author is only to offer information of a general nature to help you in your quest for emotional and spiritual well-being. This book is not meant to be used, nor should it be used, to diagnose or treat any medical condition. For diagnosis or treatment of any medical problem, consult your own physician. The author and the publisher are not responsible for any specific health needs that may require medical supervision and are not liable for any damages or negative consequences from any treatment, action, application or preparation to any person reading or following the information in this book.

ISBN: 978-0-9985346-0-2

To Carly and Max, my inspirations,
my best teachers and the lights of my life.
Without you, none of this would have been possible.

Table of Contents

Foreword

I have built a successful practice over the last 42 years by helping clients return their bodies to a state of balance, known as homeostasis, so they can heal. Essential oils can play a powerful role in helping the body achieve homeostasis as this book thoroughly explains.

Homeostasis in the body is largely maintained by our autonomic nervous system which balances the body's involuntary functions such as body temperature, heart rate and many aspects of detoxification.

This balance is maintained via bi-lateral communications between the body and the brain. Sensory nerve fibers relay information from the organs and bodily functions to the brain, and the autonomic nervous system responds by sending signals through the efferent neurons to the organs, muscles, and glandular tissues. The goal is to help keep this communication channel open and balanced.

As you may know, the autonomic nervous system has two divisions that work to counteract each other and keep the body in balance. The sympathetic division is responsible for the "fight or flight" response and prepares the body for physical exertion while its counterpart, the parasympathetic division, calms the body down and is the "rest and digest" state of being.

The body needs to return smoothly to a parasympathetic state to avoid over-stimulation that can lead to increased risk for heart conditions, depressed immune function, poor digestion and nutritional deficiencies, all of which open the door for exhausted adrenal function and auto immunity.

I have taught thousands of practitioners how to test and balance the autonomic nervous system through my proprietary system of Autonomic Response Testing to help support clients with autoimmune disorders, chronic infections, illness and pain,

We are all bio-individual, which means that external and internal stressors affect us all differently and there is no one size fits all cure. My Autonomic Response Testing system is a biofeedback enhanced physical exam which uses changes in muscle tone to identify specific stressors in each individual along with the optimal remedy or intervention to neutralize that stress response. To do so, we first determine what is stressing the body, by assessing different structural, psychological, biochemical and/ or electromagnetic stressors. We then assess the resonance of different remedies to help neutralize the stress response and return the body to the balanced state where healing, regeneration and detoxification occur.

Essential oils have become an integral part of my practice as they can be used to match the resonance of different organs and regions of the brain to help bring the body back into balance. They can also be used to activate the parasympathetic response, also called a yin state, by applying a stimulatory oil to the skin near the vagus ganglia behind the ear and can assist in helping to move lymphatic fluid.

I also believe that healing occurs on more than just the physical level. For individuals who are chronically ill, it is important to tap into what I call the five levels of healing that include:
- Physical
- Energetic
- Mental
- Intuitive
- Spiritual

Essential oils can be used to open the system to all five levels of healing. It is critical to address and heal all five levels for complete healing and lasting wellness.

On a physical level, essential oils are highly anti-bacterial, anti-microbial and anti-viral and can be used to help modulate immune reactions and calm the nervous system. For example, any given oil contains 80-300 or more different constituents. They also make wonderful transdermal remedies as the molecules in one drop of essential oils are so small they can enter the body anywhere on the skin. I have had good success using essential oils to support lymphatic movement which is so important in detoxification efforts.

Essential oils can also work on the energy body, balancing the electric currents of the body and nervous system (and the chakras), acupuncture meridians, and the biophoton field (sometimes referred to as the aura). Conventional diagnostic methods such as EKG, HRV, MRI, X-rays, and CAT scans also work on the energetic body level as do alternative diagnostic methods such as thermography, Autonomic Response Testing, kinesiology, and Chinese pulses. Other treatments that work on the energy body include acupuncture, Qigong, meditation, breath therapy, bodywork, yoga, microcurrent therapies, and radiation treatments.

Essential Oils are particularly well suited to support healing of the mental body, where your life experiences are recorded as thoughts, beliefs, emotions and attitudes. This book does an excellent job explaining how and why essential oils can be used to help release mental thought patterns. Other energetic modalities that can work to heal on this deep level include Mental Field Therapy (MFT), homeopathy, Applied Psycho-Neurobiology (APN), and psychotherapy.

Essential oils can also amplify healing in the intuitive body, also known as the "transpersonal human energy field", or simply our connection with others. This level of healing can also be supported with diagnostic methods and healing techniques such as APN, dream analysis, art therapy, color and sound therapies, hypnotherapy, Shamanism, Jungian Psychotherapy, and Systemic Family Constellations.

The fifth level of healing, your spirit body, is unique to your relationship with your God, spirit or higher consciousness.

Essential oils have long history in religious ceremony as they can be used to help amplify this consciousness in combination with personal prayer, chanting or meditation.

While essential oils can be used simply to treat particular symptoms, Vibrant Blue Oils approach of addressing the underlying foundations to bring specific organs, including the brain, back into balance is more consistent with my approach to supporting the body to heal itself. This book provides excellent information to help you assess your health imbalances and prioritize healing protocols. In addition, Jodi's discovery that certain essential oils, when combined in specific synergistic combinations, expand their healing benefits exponentially beyond that of the individual oils, is consistent with my testing of—and working with—the Vibrant Blue Oil remedies.

I've been very impressed with the quality, unique formulation, and vibration of Vibrant Blue Oils. The remedies test strongly using ART and are a wonderful therapeutic tool for the nervous system.

Dietrich Klinghardt MD, PhD

Introduction

My discovery of essential oils began when my life hit rock bottom. It was a very challenging time. My husband was hospitalized, and I found myself on my own, working and caring for our two young children. None of us were sleeping. And we were all anxious and on edge. But I could no longer muster the energy to even get out of bed, let alone answer the phone or juggle all the responsibilities in my life.

I had so much to do, but so little physical or emotional energy. My technical diagnosis was likely adrenal exhaustion, or possibly failure, that also presented as depression. It felt like I had literally run of out gas and even the littlest things felt overwhelming. I knew I needed help, but didn't know where to find it. I had experienced an adverse reaction when I tried to use pharmaceutical drugs to alleviate my post-partum depression, so I didn't want to go that route. Sadly, I was at a loss for what else to do.

I have a degree in nutritional therapy, so I was actively working to lift my mood with herbs and supplements, with marginal success. I tried everything I could think of, including intense restrictive diets that were exhausting to implement and sustain, especially in my already depleted state, loads of expensive supplements, and all sorts of alternative therapies. Sure, they helped a little, but the underlying issues still lingered. It felt a bit like treading water—the protocols helped prevent me from drowning, but never pulled me to shore.

One day, a dear friend showed up at my doorstep and handed me a box of essential oils. "Here, these will help you," he said. When I asked how to use them, he responded, "You are very smart and very intuitive, you will figure it out." Then he left.

Lacking the energy even to get off the couch to research anything on the computer, I intuitively tested to see if one of the oils could help support my exhausted adrenal glands. (You may be familiar with applied kinesiology or "muscle testing," with which one can evaluate the body's imbalances by checking for strengths and weaknesses.) I was surprised when instead of a single oil standing out, five of them tested well. I intuitively combined them into a blend that immediately began to boost my energy, mood, and mental clarity. It was akin to what I imagine it must be like to almost drown and then come up for air. I continued to use the oils for several weeks until I began to feel like myself again.

Buoyed by my positive experience, I began exploring essential oils, experimenting with them, and mixing them into blends. I shared my creations with friends and fellow practitioners, all of whom had overwhelmingly positive experiences.

I began researching how others used essential oils. I was surprised to realize that no one was using essential oils to balance the underlying issues in the body, brain, and emotions so we can heal. In other words, others were using essential oils to treat symptoms, like a stuffy nose or poor sleep. I was discovering the ability of essential oils to bring specific organs and the brain back into balance, thereby supporting the body to heal itself.

Now I was inspired!

My recovery was so astonishing that I was deeply motivated to learn the capability of these oils—and blends especially—to improve health. I continued to create proprietary blends of organic and wildcrafted, therapeutic essential oils to support different organs in the body and regions of the brain, all of which met with powerful results. These blends laid the foundation for Vibrant Blue Oils, a company that has been offering therapeutic quality, practitioner-tested blends since 2013!

My primary intention with Vibrant Blue Oils has always been to empower my customers and personal clients with the tools and the knowledge to return their bodies to vibrant health. My intention in writing this book is to compile all the knowledge I have gleaned on why essential oils work and how to use them so that YOU can be empowered to reclaim your health.

It is my sense that current usage of essential oils merely scratches the surface of their potential. It is not dissimilar to my 87-year-old neighbor who uses his iPhone solely as a phone, to make and receive telephone calls. My children are constantly trying to teach him how to use it to take pictures, navigate directions or send and receive emails, none of which really interest him. He just wants to use it as a phone. And that usage is not incorrect. It certainly can be used just as a phone, just as essential oils can be used just to make a bath or room smell good, but that usage only scratches the surface of the potential for healing with essential oils.

A deeper potential is to use essential oils to rebalance different tissues and organs in the body. Recognizing that it is important to understand what organ is out of balance in order to heal it, I was inspired to write this book and share that knowledge. For example, one customer complained of not seeing improvement from usage of the **LIVER**™ oil. It quickly became apparent that she was using the wrong oil and would benefit more from the **GALLBLADDER**™ oil, which brought her immediate relief.

While I am not a medical doctor and have no business or intention of diagnosing, treating, curing or preventing diseases, I did spend several years working as a researcher and an award-winning journalist. Drawing on those skills to better understand my own powerful transformation with essential oils, I have dedicated half a decade to reading every book, blog, and research study I could find on essential oils and why they work. The compilation of what I learned, taking certain pieces from different sources and combining them in a way that made sense to me, is what I hope to share with YOU.

Please don't get me wrong. I am not claiming that essential oils by themselves are a magic bullet for every condition. But I do know from my clinical and personal experience that, when combined with other dietary and lifestyle modifications, they can dramatically bolster and improve your health. Now I'm passionate to share my story and knowledge with you.

It is my sincere hope that this book will help you support your own health and the health of your family, friends, or clients. For many of you, the protocols in this book may support immediate shifts in your health, vitality and energy. For others, this book may just be a starting point that helps you advance to a deeper level of healing.

Wherever you are in your healing journey, please remember that you are not alone and that you have the power to support your own vibrant health. I hope this book helps to empower you with the tools and knowledge to support you in navigating your own healing journey. I am honored to have been part of your journey, and I hope we can stay connected.

My passion for educating people on essential oils grows deeper with every new discovery, success story and every client who challenges me to research more solutions. I love to connect with readers to learn about successes and challenges they have faced and to share the latest research and clinical feedback in essential oils, so let's stay in touch. You can find me on social media and by visiting my website—www.vibrantblueoils.com/bookbonus—for access to the latest updates. I hope to see you there!

In vibrant health,

Jodi Cohen
www.vibrantblueoils.com
www.facebook.com/vibrantblueoils

Chapter 1

Why Essential Oils Work

Essential oils are the natural, highly concentrated essences extracted from plants, shrubs, flowers, fruits, bushes, roots, bark or trees in their living state for their healing capabilities.

The plants from which essential oils are derived have been used for medicinal purposes throughout history. In fact, most of our modern drugs are plants that have been modified enough to secure a patent (no natural substance can be patented). Some 50% of the pharmaceutical drugs produced during the last thirty years are either directly or indirectly derived from plant medicine. For example, the pain-relieving and anti-inflammatory effects of aspirin mimic the chemical compound salicin found in white willow bark. Similarly, Valium (Diazepam) is a synthetic analog to the herb valerian root.

Humans have long consumed plants for their healing value. Many popular healing diets consist primarily of food from organic plants and the ethically raised animals that feed on those plants. An extremely successful example of the healing power of plants can be attributed to Dr. Terry Wahls who recovered from MS by eating specific plants that feed our mitochondria, the energy generators in our cells. Wahls recommends a diet that includes a daily dose of nine cups of plants to boost our body's ability to make the energy necessary to heal.

Plants, and the highly concentrated essences of plants that are distilled into essential oils, can be used to compliment and support whole food healing diets and lifestyle protocols. They can help us digest and assimilate nutrients, heal the gut, support organs of detoxification, relax the adrenals, reduce negative thought patterns and support sleep.

What's more, essential oils can support healing in an easy to absorb, topically applied or inhaled form that even young children or those with digestive challenges, or contra indication to medicine can tolerate and assimilate.

Why Do Essential Oils Work?

Essential oils provide the key components of the plants' immune systems. They help the plants grow, thrive, evolve, and adapt to their surroundings. For example, they protect plants from bacterial and viral infections, heal injuries, repel unwanted predators and other environmental damage, and help deliver nutrients to the cells. This makes them "essential" for a plant as they help the plants survive.

Essential oils play a similar role in the human body, perhaps due to our shared chemistry. Both essential oils and humans are made of three primary elements—carbon, hydrogen, and oxygen—which make essential oils highly compatible with human biochemistry.

Research has shown that essential oils help us fight infection (with antibacterial, antifungal, and antiviral properties), balance hormones and emotions, and aid in regeneration.

Essential Oils: The Back Door to Optimal Health

The front door for carrying healing nutrients and energy into the body is our digestive system. When it is working optimally, we can digest, absorb, and assimilate all the nutrients we need and efficiently eliminate all waste products.

Unfortunately, the cumulative damage of processed foods, GMOs, chemically treated water, environmental toxins, and increased stress have impeded the optimal function of many people's digestive systems, leading to a range of health challenges, including fatigue, weight gain, brain fog, and pain.

We know that if digestion is compromised, or the road of the digestive track into the body is partially blocked, it can be challenging to assimilate nutrients through that channel. This is one of the reasons that many people continually test low for nutrients like vitamin D, vitamin B, zinc, or iron despite frequent supplementation. The digestive track is not working properly and therefore not assimilating nutrients via oral consumption.

But the good news is that even though the front door to healing—the digestive system—is partially blocked or closed, the body does have some back doors to access the system.

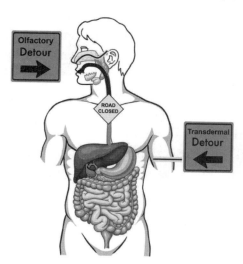

These back doors are the olfactory system and the skin. Essential oils are uniquely suited to open these back doors, accessing your body through your skin and your olfactory system when the front door of your digestive system is impaired and not able to optimally assimilate and absorb healing nutrients. And these back doors may be able to access your body more powerfully and effectively than can your digestive tract.

You see, your sense of smell (part of your olfactory system), is one of the most powerful channels into the body. The sense of smell is uniquely able to directly access the limbic system, an area of your brain where you store emotions and long-term memory. This direct access is the easiest way for you to release fear and anger-based thought patterns that keep your body locked into a stressed state.

And you won't believe how quickly it works! The entire process from the initial inhalation of an essential oil to a corresponding response in the body can happen in a matter of seconds.

Similarly, your skin, which is your largest organ, is relatively permeable to fat-soluble substances like essential oils. The molecules of essential oils are so small that they can pass through your skin into the capillaries and quickly be absorbed into the bloodstream. From there, they can disperse to specific organs. One study found that the constituents of topically applied lavender oil were measurable in the blood within twenty minutes, and they stayed in the blood system for up to ninety minutes.

Finally, because of the ease of administration, essential oils are ideal for anyone with compromised digestion, who might be taking medications that contraindicate supplements, who struggle to find natural alternatives that are vegan or gluten-free, or for children who struggle with swallowing supplements.

Inhalation

Our sense of smell, which is part of our olfactory system, is one of the most powerful channels into the body. It allows us to detect the subtlest fragrance over a great distance. The scent of Vanilla, for instance, can be detected even in low concentrations of 0.00000000762 grains per cubic inch.

Research further confirms that inhalation can be the most direct and effective method for using essential oils. When we inhale essential oils through the nose, the odor molecules trigger receptor sites in our mucous membrane, which then sends the odor information on to the olfactory bulb, which is located at the top and on both sides of the inner nasal cavity, approximately at eye level.

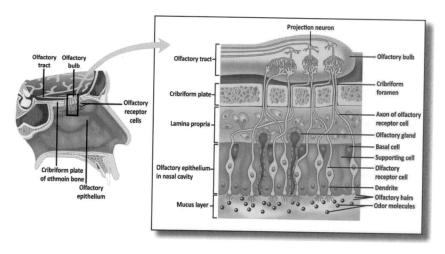

The olfactory bulb is covered with a mucous membrane, known as the olfactory epithelium, which is lined on both sides with a special tissue consisting of about ten million olfactory nerve cells covered with a layer of mucus. These nerve cells are replaced every twenty-eight days.

Each nerve cell carries a bundle consisting of six to eight tiny hairs or cilia equipped with receptor cells. The hairs attached to the nerve cells—up to eighty million of them—are capable of carrying a tremendous amount of information, a capability that outperforms every known analytical human function.

The cells of the olfactory epithelium are in fact brain cells. This olfactory membrane is the only place in the human body where the central nervous system is exposed and is in direct contact with the environment!

Odor molecules stimulate tiny hair bundles carried by nerve cells in the form of electrical impulses. The minute extensions at the site of the nerve bundles are located in the nasal cavity where they pass through the ethmoid bone behind the septum to the brain. There they come in contact with the olfactory bulb, which in turn passes along the stimulus to the relevant location in the brain.

Fragrant substances pass on to the limbic system without being registered by the cerebral cortex. From there, they reach the innermost control centers in the brain.

It is not the essential oil itself that is sent to the brain, but a neural translation of the oils. These fragrance messages are interpreted and transmitted to the limbic system of the brain, known as the "emotional brain" because it deals with emotional and psychological responses.

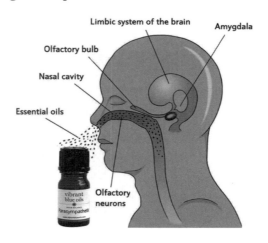

As you may know, the limbic system serves as the control center in the brain for emotions and feelings, along with hunger, thirst, and sex drive. This helps explain how scent can influence appetite and sexual attraction. It also impacts long-term memory through the hippocampus, which stores our memories. The hippocampus is the area of the brain at play during those powerful experiences when smell triggers a particular emotion or memory. Who hasn't sensed a particular aroma and been transported back through time to the memory of a particular person or event? For me, the mere smell of mothballs transports me back in time to my grandparents' apartment in Brooklyn, triggering a multisensory memory including both the visuals and the emotions that I experienced during our annual visits.

This powerful emotional reaction in the limbic system is triggered by nerve impulses which, in turn, trigger other areas of the brain that are responsible for secreting hormones and neurotransmitters and for regulating body functions. For example, the pituitary gland releases endorphins, which can help alleviate pain and promote a sense of well-being. In fact, essential oils may stimulate or sedate the brain to promote or inhibit the production and release of various neurotransmitters, which then impact the nervous system.

This makes essential oils especially powerful tools for dealing with emotional challenges, like anxiety, depression, fear, worry, grief, trauma, anger, and self-abuse. As you may know, emotions and thought patterns could trigger an ongoing stress response in the body (since our stress response cannot differentiate between physical or emotional and thought-driven stressors) that impedes our ability to heal. Smelling essential oils can be a powerful tool for moving through and releasing these thought patterns.

Topical Application

Topical, or transdermal, applications allow active ingredients of healing substances to be delivered across the skin for systemic distribution to different organs, like the liver, gallbladder, pancreas, or adrenals. This transdermal application offers an effective alternative to oral delivery and serves as a backdoor channel to stimulate different organs or regions of the brain.

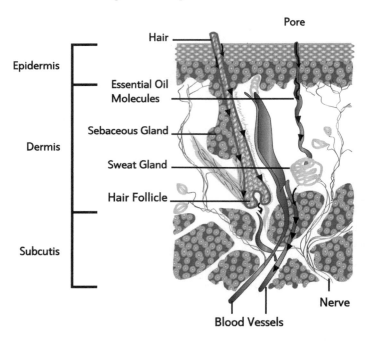

As you may know, the brain needs oxygen, glucose, and stimulation to function. This stimulation can come in the form of stimulatory essential oils. For example, stimulatory oils, like Vibrant Blue Oils **PARASYMPATHETIC**™ blend, can be topically applied behind the earlobe and up one inch on the mastoid bone to stimulate the vagal nerve—the on/off switch between the "rest-and-digest" parasympathetic state of the nervous system and the sympathetic "fight-or-flight" state.

The skin is our largest organ and is relatively permeable to fat-soluble substances like essential oils. For thousands of years, people have placed healing substances on the skin for therapeutic effects. Modern medicine has taken advantage of this transdermal channel, developing a variety of topical formulations to treat local indications. Consider the use of patches for motion sickness, nicotine addiction, contraception, and hormone replacement.

This topical delivery channel has a variety of advantages compared with the oral route, especially as it can bypass the stomach and liver, both of which can chemically alter the therapeutic effects of drugs and essential oils.

Also, topical application is non-invasive and easy to administer. For example, you can apply specific blends over the organ systems they are designed to balance for optimal results. To balance anxiety or fatigue, which is often a reflection of underlying adrenal imbalances, you might apply indicated essential oils, like ADRENAL™, on the lower back over the adrenal glands.

Internal Ingestion

I do not recommend ingesting essential oils. Several studies show that taking essential oils internally is, in fact, the least effective way to absorb their therapeutic properties. The oil often winds up in the digestive tract where it has to pass through the stomach and the small intestine before it reaches the bloodstream. This process can chemically alter the essential oils and can be toxic to the liver or the kidneys. And remember, the front door of the digestive system is often compromised, so why would you want to inhibit the effectiveness of these powerful healing remedies?

I have talked to many people who claim benefits from internal consumption of essential oils. However, when I dig deeper, I find most of them are adding the oils to water and drinking it. As you drink the water, you inhale the essential oils, so it is likely through the olfactory channel, not the digestive tract, that the oils and their benefits are being assimilated into the body. And it could be that the oils are being absorbed more directly into the bloodstream through the highly sensitive capillaries in the mouth, bypassing the digestive tract.

I have found topical applications to be far more effective. For example, oils touted for internal use of digestive distress, like peppermint oil, or Vibrant Blue Oils **INTESTINAL MUCOSA**™, can also produce the same results when topically massaged over the small intestine.

Why Essential Oils Work

There are many theories on why essential oils work. I believe it is a combination of:

> ➤ The ability of essential oils to return the body to **homeostasis**
> ➤ The unique **chemistry** of essential oils
> ➤ The ability to **cross the blood-brain barrier**
> ➤ The **healing value of plants** in both our food and concentrated in essential oils
> ➤ The **farm-to-table** process of distilling oils immediately after they are picked to capture the nutrients at the height of their vitality

Supporting the Body's Homeostasis

Our bodies continually toggle in and out of balance. When we respond to any physical or emotional stress, our bodies release stress hormones that cause our breathing to increase, our heart to beat faster, and our blood to flow to external muscles and away from the digestive organs. All of these responses allow us to flee from a pressing emergency. When the stressful situation passes, our breathing and heart rate return to normal. This ability to return to balance is known as homeostasis. It is in this balanced state that our body can rest, repair, and heal.

This balance also exists in nature. We know that the tides, the seasons, the circadian rhythm of day and night, along with the cycles of the moon all ebb and flow in balance. Our bodies are designed to maintain a similar natural rhythm.

This is one reason that connecting to nature through the consumption of nutrient-dense whole food, hiking in the woods, walking barefoot on the grass or dirt, or relaxing by the water is so healing. We allow our bodies to align with the natural rhythm of the planet. When we lose this connection to nature, it interferes with our internal rhythm and balance, impeding our ability to return to balance so we can relax, sleep, detoxify, digest, repair, and heal.

When our bodies are in the balanced state of homeostasis, these natural processes flow easily without interference. The body can easily recognize and respond to a stressor, then return to balance.

I love the analogy that when a plane flies between two destinations, it does not fly on a direct path, but rather makes a small series of constant corrections to maintain its course. I believe that is ideally how the body works as well: it responds to an emotional, physical, or psychological stressor and then returns to balance.

Stresses are supposed to be short and quick so that the body can return to alignment equally quickly. Unfortunately, the chronic and prolonged stress that most of us face on a regular basis throw us so far out of balance that it becomes difficult to return to homeostasis. Disease is most likely to set in when the body is in an imbalanced state.

Connecting with nature—either by consuming nutrient-dense whole foods or inhaling or topically applying essential oils derived from plants—allows us to align with the health-supporting properties of nature so our bodies can return to balance and heal.

The definition of balance is to "maintain a steady state to avoid falling"—falling into ill health, negative thoughts, depressed or anxious mood. As our thoughts shift, so does our balance. But nature remains steady. Plants, trees, rocks—their energy remains grounded and constant.

Thus, when we align ourselves with that grounded energy of nature, it can help us return to and stay in balance. Essential oils and the energy of nature, especially oils from grounded plants like trees or grasses, help ground us and return our bodies to the state of balance and enhance our ability to change in response to the body's demands.

The Chemistry of Oils

The molecular structures of essential oils are ring-like and far more complex than the simpler, linear carbon-hydrogen structures of fatty oils. The essential oil chains are held together by carbon atoms linked with oxygen and hydrogen, along with nitrogen and sulfur atoms (which are not found in other non-essential plant oils).

It is interesting that no two essential oils are alike in their molecular structure. Each oil is comprised of a combination of hundreds—even thousands—of different natural chemicals. The average essential oil may contain anywhere from eighty to four hundred known chemical constituents, making them ideal for killing and preventing the spread of bacteria.

By way of comparison, synthetic antibiotics often contain only one active chemical, which allows bacteria (like MRSA) to mutate to survive an immune response. The large and varied numbers of antiseptic and antibacterial constituents in essential oils make it impossible for bacteria to mutate enough to survive each and every one. This is what makes essential oils such effective natural antibiotics.

The chemistry and therapeutic potential of essential oils are a direct result of how and where they are grown, harvested, and processed. To ensure optimal quality, essential oils need to be grown organically in their indigenous climate and carefully harvested, extracted, and distilled without any additives or adulterants.

Essential Oils Can Cross the Blood-Brain Barrier

The blood-brain barrier is the barrier membrane between the circulating blood and the brain. This membrane prevents certain damaging substances from reaching brain tissue and cerebrospinal fluid while allowing essential molecules to enter.

The blood-brain barrier is like a sieve or filter through which only molecules of a certain size or smaller can penetrate. The molecules of essential oils are so small that most of them can pass through the blood-brain barrier. It is interesting to note that these small molecules of essential oils make them so aromatic. The only way something can be aromatic is for the molecules to be so small that they readily leap from the surface of the substance and circulate in the air so they can enter our noses and be detected as odor and smell.

How Essential Oils Cross the Blood Brain Barrier

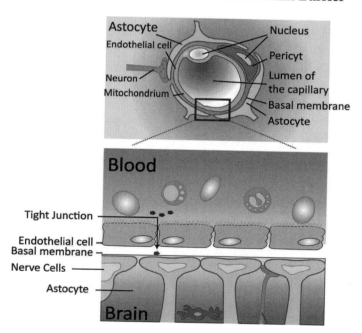

To better understand aromatic oils, you might consider that oils pressed from seeds, like corn, peanut, safflower, walnut, almond, olive, are not aromatic. Sure, they have a smell, but you can't smell them across the room in minutes (or seconds) as you can when you open a bottle of peppermint or other essential oil.

Similarly, most of the molecules of the substances used in chemotherapy are too large to pass through the blood-brain barrier, which is why doctors have found that traditional chemotherapy doesn't work on brain cancer.

Because they can cross the blood-brain barrier, essential oils can access and balance certain parts of the brain that control how your body works. The brain orchestrates your nervous system, hormones, thought processes, and memory. Dysfunction in specific parts of the brain can contribute to physical, mental, emotional, psychological, learning or behavioral problems. The ability to reset these specific regions of the brain can, therefore, improve your mental, physical, and emotional health.

The ability to cross the blood-brain barrier is often attributed to the chemistry of the oils, specifically, those that fall into the class of "terpenes", a family of molecules small enough to penetrate the blood-brain barrier. Terpenes are a class of essential oils composed of "isoprene units" or organic compounds of five connected carbon atoms with some hydrogens attached.

The terpene family includes Phenylpropanoids (only one isoprene unit), Monoterpenes (two isoprene units), Sesquiterpenes (three isoprene units), Diterpenes (four isoprene units), as well as Triterpenes (six isoprene units) and Tetrapenes (eight isoprene units).

Terpenes are found in most essential oils and are chemically credited with the ability to reprogram the DNA at a cellular level, in effect working as stem cells to correct bad cellular codes. Sesquiterpene molecules—found in Cedarwood, Vetiver, Spikenard, Sandalwood, Black Pepper, Patchouli, Myrrh, Ginger,

Galbanum, and Frankincense—are also attributed with the capability of carrying oxygen into human tissue.

I share this with you, not to overwhelm you with complex scientific information, but to demonstrate unequivocally the power of these oils to impact health. I also want you to appreciate the value of what you are learning here and to acknowledge your commitment to using essential oils responsibly. Their impact goes far beyond flavoring your water or making a room smell nice.

The Healing Potential of Plants

Plants have incredibly healing capabilities as both food and concentrated extractions such as essential oils and flower essences.

Up until very recent modern history, this was common knowledge. Humans knew how to utilize plants to heal the body. It is interesting that, in nature, wherever a harmful plant element exists, the cure is right nearby. For example, the sting of nettles can be calmed by rubbing the spores from the underside of a neighboring fern on the irritated skin. Country doctors knew how to use garlic, lemon, cayenne pepper and apple cider vinegar to heal most ailments. In our grandparents lifetime, country doctors and their knowledge have been replaced by pharmaceutical solutions.

But most of our modern drugs just mimic plant medicine with minor modifications to secure a patent (no natural substance can be patented). While plants are totally bio-familiar with humans and thus interact seamlessly, their pharmaceutical cousins, while offering primary beneficial effects, may also create undesirable side effects. That is why many drugs produce side effects, while the plant version often does not.

Bio-Familiarity between Plants and Humans

We know that people grow and thrive with a combination of sunlight, connecting to the ground (also called Grounding or Earthing) and the air (hence the benefit of deep, slow, rhythmic breathing as that allows us to absorb more life force energy than by short, shallow breathing). Plants are no different. If you think about how plants grow, firmly rooted in the earth and nourished by air and sunlight, it makes perfect sense that they would store up abundant earth energy. This is energy that they pass on to us when we consume them.

In *Aromatherapy for the Soul: Healing the Spirit with Fragrance and Essential Oils*, Valerie Ann Worwood notes, "Plants take the energy of the sun and transform it, through photosynthesis, into the food energy upon which all animals rely. Essential oils are the concentrated form of that sun energy."

An interaction with time and water makes plants more bio-available. For example, soaking and sprouting nuts and grains or fermenting vegetables make the nutrients more accessible to the body. Soaking plants in alcohol, water, glycerin or apple cider vinegar allows the nutrients to be released into tinctures that the body can absorb more effectively. The same is true for essential oils.

It is popular to talk about essential oils as an isolated substance, detailing the history of the oils or the chemistry of the oils. We may forget that these oils are the concentrated essences of our old friends, plants. These plants, especially when made more bio-available as essential oils, can have profound healing qualities. The body, when given the correct raw materials, will get into balance and heal itself. These plants are powerful tools for shifting the body into balance so healing can begin.

Layering Oils with Other Modalities

Plants in combination can also help enhance diets and supplements. It is fairly common to find that the combination of two things is so much better than an individual piece on its own. There are numerous examples from food (think ham and cheese, peanut butter and jelly, bagels and cream cheese) to music, friendships and romantic relationships.

I have been noticing the same thing with supplements and oils. Sometimes if you test a supplement on its own, it will not test well, but if you combine it with another supplement or an essential oil, the combination can put the whole system into balance.

For example, I long noticed a pattern where the combination of kelp with an iodine supplement was more powerful than either by itself. There is something about the frequency of the sea minerals in the sea kelp that activates and unlocks the nutrients in the iodine in a way that just iodine alone does not. The same holds true when combining essential oils with a nutrient-dense whole food diet and/or supplements.

The frequency of the oils seems to enhance and optimize the impact of the other nutrients. Every cell of our body vibrates. This is often referred to as the frequency of the body. Every organ and region of the brain has its own optimal frequency. These frequencies are influenced by internal and external factors including the food we eat, the external frequencies we are exposed to (like pollution and EMFs), the energy of the people we surround ourselves with and the thoughts and emotions we experience. For example, exercise is known to raise frequency because it increases respiration and heart rate. When you combine exercise with a clean diet or essential oils, the sum of the combined elements are often greater than the parts. Similarly, when you layer essential oils and a healing bath, (with Epsom salt and baking soda) it amplifies the benefits of both.

Resonance and Dissonance

This combination of like things is known as "resonance", where you match and enhance a positive frequency to bring an unhealthy organ into balance. The counterpart to resonance is known as dissonance, or canceling out a harmful frequency as in the case of inflammation. Essential oils blends can serve both functions in the body, amplifying the positive or minimizing the negative.

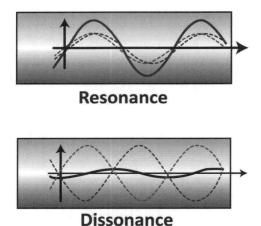

Resonance

Dissonance

To prove the point, have your practitioner test a supplement alone and then with a combination of a particular Vibrant Blue Oil and the same supplement. When I have done this with clients, I find the combination always trumps the supplement alone. The Vibrant Blue Oil **PARASYMPATHETIC**™ blend seems to be particularly effective at boosting the benefit of a particular supplement.

Benefits of Eating Seasonally and Organically

There is much research on the value of eating seasonally and organically, known as farm to table, as the nutritional value slowly begins to decline as food decays. If we can consume our food shortly after it has been harvested, either in a farm-to-table setting or at a local farmer's market, it packs a stronger nutritional punch than food that has been shipped across the country, or across the world, prior to consumption.

In his book *Medical Medium*, Anthony Williams heralds the benefits of eating unwashed produce straight from the earth with the film of life still on it to bolster our health. Dr. Richard Bach, who created Bach Flower Essences, also believed that the dew found on flower petals holds the plant's healing energy and that energy is especially effective for healing emotional and spiritual conditions.

While we often cannot consume our produce the day it is picked, essential oils are often distilled on the spot within hours of harvesting, capturing the chemical constituents and nutrients at the height of their vitality.

In his book *Aveda Rituals: A Daily Guide to Natural Beauty and Health*, Horst Rechelbacher, the founder of the Aveda Corporation, notes that essential oils are created by "pressing and distilling them in water while they are in full bloom, extracting the life energy they contain and preserving them in liquid form. Although the plant soon dies, its biological information stays alive in the form of an essence as long as the essence is kept fresh, away from light and heat."

Because of their unique molecular structures, different distillation and extraction techniques are required to draw essences from different plants and flowers. For instance, most plants can be distilled with steam or water; they weigh less than water and therefore, float on top of the water solution until they naturally separate. Citrus fruits need to be cold pressed because the essential oils are located in little sacs just under the surface of the peel and need to be pressed out. Some oils, like jasmine, cannot be distilled and need to be extracted directly from the bloom using a process called Enfleurage, where a fatty substance is used to extract the oils. Almost all of our Vibrant Blue Oils are distilled using low temperature and low-pressure steam distillation.

All of these natural, non-invasive methods of immediate extraction help preserve the chemical constituents and nutrients of the oils.

Essential Oils are Highly Concentrated

It is also important to note that essential oils are highly concentrated, making them even more potent carriers of the healing essence of the plants. An entire plant, when distilled, might produce only a single drop of essential oil. This makes essential oils approximately seventy-five to one hundred times more concentrated, and consequently far more potent, than dried herbs. This potency can be used to activate or amplify the healing benefit of foods, supplements, or dried herbs taken in combination with essential oils. As I mentioned, I have long observed that the oils help to activate and enhance the nutrients in the supplements for better absorption and assimilation.

Because they are so concentrated, it is important to ensure that oils are grown without toxins like pesticides, chemical fertilizers, adulterants or added synthetic chemicals that would then be concentrated during the distillation process. For example, Vibrant Blue Oils essential oils are either certified organic, organically grown in countries that do not offer organic certification, or wild crafted in nature.

Oils are Programmable

If we think of essential oils as "living energy," it is important to consider how our various actions and thoughts determine the effectiveness of the oils. Like stem cells, they can be programmed both by their unique chemistry and the intent with which they are blended and applied.

This is because essential oils have electrical properties, which are subject to our thoughts and feelings. It is interesting that the same essential oil will have different effects on different people. It could be that because individuals have distinct chemistries, the same oil will have a different chemical effect on each.

I also believe thought and intent are key factors. We are aware of the "mind-body connection"—thought and intent affect our physiology. Essential oils can amplify this intent. Our intent in creating and blending the oils is to balance specific organs and regions of the brain. Your intent in applying the oils can amplify their healing value. As you apply the oil, if you send thoughts of love to the organ or a particular region of the brain and instruct that part of the body to return to balance, you will amplify the healing potential.

I was very skeptical of this until I looked at research performed that looked at how intent and prayer modified the crystalline structure of water.

In his book, *The Hidden Messages from Water*, Japanese scientist Masaru Emoto, graphically demonstrated how different thought, intention, and emotional energies alter the crystalline structure of frozen water.

His research focused on how "negative" and "positive" words would affect the water. He placed water over cards with positive words like "love," "angel," or "appreciation" written on them. He then crystallized the water. Examining the crystals under a microscope, he observed light, beautiful icy patterns. He repeated the experiment using negative words like "hate," "demon," or "kill." The water samples associated with negative energies produced dark, ugly, malformed crystals.

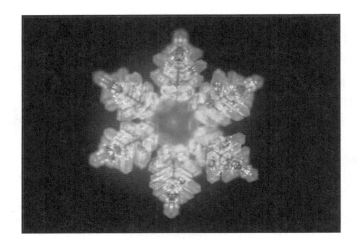

Photo of Water Crystal formed after exposure to the word "Truth"
(C) Office Masaru Emoto, LLC

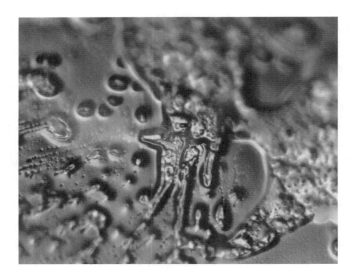

Photo of Water Crystal formed after exposure to the words "You Disgust Me"
(C) Office Masaru Emoto, LLC

Similarly, in the 1950s a researcher named Franklin Loehr explored the effect of prayer and human thought on water, which he details in *The Power of Prayer on Plants*. The two hydrogen atoms in a water molecule are attached to the single oxygen atom at specific angles which can range from 110–120 degrees. Loehr found that human thought alters the bonding angles between the oxygen and hydrogen atoms, thus changing the physical properties of the water.

Like water and plants, research shows that essential oils also respond to words, thoughts, and prayer and even amplify each other. In some of essential oil researcher Bruce Tainio's work, the frequency of essential oils were measured before and after being bombarded with positive or negative thoughts.

Frequency is a measurable rate of electrical energy that is constant between any two points. Our bodies are electrical, and everything around us has electrical frequencies. Essential oils have a coherent, harmonic frequency, so they are harmonious with the electrical field of the human body.

Tainio found that positive thoughts aimed at the oils raised their frequencies by 10 MHz and prayer increased their frequencies by 15 MHz. The opposite is also true as negative thoughts drove frequencies down by 12 MHz.

Power of Intent

Essential oils work to amplify intent on many levels, including physical, mental, emotional, social, and spiritual. They can balance the organs and regions of the brain, moving molecules of oils to where they can best serve to heal the body. Their vibrations resonate with the tissues in helpful ways, according to our wishes and mental directions. They also work in the limbic systems to help clear negative feelings and blocked emotions, thus eliminating the root causes of many diseases and conditions

In *The Chemistry of Essential Oils*, David Stewart writes, "Chemistry determines what is possible. Our thoughts won't change the chemistry of an oil; that is fixed before we apply the oil. But our thoughts can determine which aspects of the chemistry will work in our bodies."

An intent for balancing and healing the body may be imbued throughout the process of growing, harvesting, distilling, blending, packaging, and distributing essential oils. For this reason, it is important to source oils that have been handled with positive intent, as plants and oils that are treated with love are charged with greater healing properties.

It would make sense that essential oils from plants grown in the same area should have the same chemical makeup, but this is often not the case. We often find plants grown on the small family farm almost always have a higher level of positive healing energy associated with them compared to oils that are grown on large industrialized plantations. We feel this is simply due to the love and caring energies the small farmers instill into the soil and the plants. (It is this intention and love that I imbue in all the Vibrant Blue Oils blends.)

It is your responsibility to consciously participate in enhancing that intent with your application of the product. The oils are powerful healing tools and will work without any participation from you when you apply them. But their healing properties will also be enhanced with your participation.

For example, when an oil is applied to any part of the body you can mentally direct it to go to wherever it is needed and affirm the outcome you desire. Your affirmation must be more than a one-time thought, but must come from within your deepest convictions and faith and be repeated and consciously retained until the desired results are manifested.

Chapter 2

How to Use Essential Oils

I t has been my observation that many essential oil companies, in discussing the characteristics and accompanying benefits of their various essential oils, describe properties similar to those offered by pharmaceutical drugs. These companies extoll the symptoms a particular oil or blend addresses, albeit in a more natural way, but they never explain how the oils might address the underlying imbalance that is causing the issue.

I believe essential oils can have the greatest impact helping people not only manage, but tackle and rebalance the underlying issue. I have found that this can be accomplished through synergistic blends that help align and balance the organs of the body and regions of the brain for optimal healing.

Addressing the Underlying Health Imbalances

When I first started working with essential oils, I was struck by the potential to utilize them in tandem with dietary and lifestyle modifications to address the root issues that throw the body out of balance and make it challenging to rest, repair, regenerate, and heal.

Most health issues can be traced to imbalances in the organs and regions of the brain associated with the following systems:

➢ Sleep
➢ Stress
➢ Digestion
➢ Gut inflammation, which is often at the root of systemic inflammation, along with mental focus and mood challenges.
➢ Blood sugar balance
➢ Detoxification support
➢ Circulation

If you can return the organs, systems or region of the brain to balance, the body can usually return to homeostasis and begin the process of healing. These inroads can, of course, be made with diet and lifestyle modifications. Essential oils add a little additional support to help expedite the journey.

Combining Essential Oils into Blends

Essential oils are extremely powerful as single oils, but there is something about combining single oils into blends that both amplifies and enhances the healing power of the oils. It is almost like a good marriage or friendship—the synergy of the two energies combined significantly enhances both individuals.

You might think of single oils like individual instruments: a blend is more like a symphony where the single oils respond to each other and adjust their individual frequencies to form a harmonious, coherent, functional blend designed to serve a particular function, like balancing an organ system or region of the brain.

A single oil not commonly associated with a specific organ may work so well in a blend because a compound acting alone can behave very differently in the balanced environment of an essential oil blend. In *The Chemistry of Essential Oils Made Simple*, David Stewart writes that single oils can "adjust their vibrations to play in harmony with the rest of the family of compounds that define the blend."

Stewart further notes that essential oil blends "resonate with body tissues at the frequencies intrinsic to their molecular spectrum as well as their resultant harmonic and beat frequencies. This increases your natural electromagnetic vibrations and restores coherence to your electric fields to produce healing and maintain wellness." He suggests that "we should maintain a certain level and spectrum of harmonic vibrations within our body to maintain health. When our electromagnetic frequencies fall below certain levels, we become susceptible to colds and flu." We know that our lifestyle choices can support optimal health, including the quality of the food we eat, our thoughts, and our emotions. Positive thoughts and emotions, like those of love, joy, and peace elevate our health, while negative thoughts and emotions like anxiety, resentment, jealousy, and depression can bring us down. I find it interesting that Stewart credits essential oils as possessing the highest and most coherent measured frequencies of all natural substances.

Another viable theory, put forth by Essential Oils expert Robert Tisserand in his Therapeutic Foundations of Essential Oils Course, is that synergy could occur because the constituents of one oil may help the constituents of another oil penetrate through the cell membrane so the results are more effective.

I believe this is why, when several single essential oils are synergistically combined for a specific healing intention, the result is often more powerful than the sum of its parts. The combination yields not only the power of the combined chemical constituents but also the synergy of how they interact together. This means that the respective powers of the individual oils change to enhance their energy. For example, the anti-inflammatory effects of chamomile are increased when combined with lavender.

The Exponential Power of Blends

The power of these essential oil synergies was thoroughly explored and explained by a medical doctor from Dallas named Jerry Tennant. In his book *Healing is Voltage*, Tennant hypothesized that the human body is like a computer. Our hardware is our structure and cells, produced from the food and nutrients we consume. Our software is the genetic code or blueprint that differentiates a liver cell from a brain cell.

If you think about it, we all start out as stem cells but somehow the body knows to follow a clear blueprint or code to differentiate the cells in the body to perform different functions. Biologist Rupert Sheldrake writes about these biological blueprints, which he called "morphic fields" in his book, *The Presence of the Past: Morphic Resonance and the Habits of Nature*.

Tennant theorizes that there is a frequency or code that instructs cells in the body to perform different functions, just as software code in a computer allows Excel and Word to perform different functions.

And just like computer software programs get viruses, our cell software can get viruses in the form of cancer or autoimmune conditions. Tennant hypothesizes that just as computer software code can be repaired and rebooted, the body's software code can also be repaired and rebooted.

Tennant believes that essential oils can be combined into blends to match the blueprint of healthy organs and therefore repair and reboot the software code of the body. It's a little bit like the idea of stem cells—they have not yet been programmed, so they carry the blueprint of healthy organ tissue and bring the body back into balance. Essential oils can play a similar role, aligning the organs of the body with the blueprint of healthy organ tissue so that the body can return to balance and heal.

How Essential Oils Reboot the Body

Since humans and plants are bio-familiar, or biologically familiar to each other, Tennant hypothesizes they use the same software codes, which he calls frequencies, with each plant having a unique frequency, much as you would perceive a unique color or musical note. Just as you can combine musical notes and instruments to make beautiful harmonies or combine paint colors to match a specific hue, you can mix the frequencies of different plants through the use of their oils to match the frequency or code of a particular organ, region of the brain, or emotional energy in balance. Topically applying this blueprint of the organ in balance can help to shift the body back into balance.

David Stewart expresses a similar view in *The Chemistry of Essential Oils Made Simple*, noting that molecules of essential oils resonate with your tissues at the frequency of healthy tissue, which restores the organ to its natural, healthy state.

Stewart explains that when opera singers shatter crystal, it is because of a principle known as resonance, where two things vibrate in unison, in essence, matching frequencies. If the opera singer could perfectly match the tone of a piece of crystal, the glass would break. It was the resonance that shattered the glass, not just volume. If he sang a note that did not match the frequency of the crystal, the glass would not shatter, no matter how loudly he sang.

"Essential oils work in a similar fashion. The various organs, tissues, and cells of your body inherently possess certain pitches or fundamental frequencies. Oil molecules that resonate at the frequency of your pancreas will administer therapy there," according to Stewart.

Swiss researcher Hans Jenny found that each organ in the body makes sound at specific frequencies. The sound is not audible to the human ear, but the vibrations of the sound are measurable. Jenny found that when an organ malfunctions, it no longer emits the healthy sound frequency. He then employed the principal of resonance; aiming specific, audible, high-intensity frequencies of sound at the organ, he could, in essence, reboot the organ and return it to health. As Stewart explains, "the sick organs were out of tune and in a state of dissonance. By coming into a place of resonance with the healthy (sound) frequencies," they would return to balance and health. That is what essential oils do. That is how they work—by resonance with organs, cells, and even our thoughts and emotions.

This is where the true potential of essential oils lies: in using them to reboot different organs or regions of the brain to return to balance. Much as you might reboot your phone or computer when glitches appear, essential oil blends that match the frequency of healthy organs and regions of the brain can be inhaled or topically applied to return the body to homeostasis, in essence rebooting our body's computer.

You might think of it as a floatation device or spotting a child as they learn a new skill. A good example is the process of teaching a child to ride a bike. In effect, you are supporting the child as you balance the bike and propel the child forward, all in the effort to help the child feel the balance in his or her body. Once the child internalizes that sense of balance, he or she can take off on his or her own.

The oils provide a similar floatation-device-like support, keeping the organ in balance and helping to repair the code until the body can remember how to maintain its own balance without the external support. That is one of the reasons I intentionally use only 5 ml bottles. The oils work quickly to shift organs; you don't use them in perpetuity, just as you wouldn't continue to take aspirin after a headache is gone.

Prioritizing Health Concerns

One key to healing is balancing the body in order of priority. This means treating the issue that the body deems most important. For example, many clients suffer from intestinal permeability. While it is important to heal this condition, it is also important to look at the underlying cause of the condition and treat that as well. Chronic and prolonged stress or poor sleep habits can compromise the ability of the gut to heal. While healing diets and supplemental protocols can be effective in the short term, the condition will often return until you address and heal the underlying condition.

Key Health Priorities

Sleep: If you struggle to fall asleep or stay asleep, it can often throw off all other systems, as sleep is the key time for the body to rest and repair. Often just improving sleep patterns can pave the way for improved blood sugar balance, detoxification, digestion, and health.

Stress: Stress is defined as any reaction to a physical, emotional, psychological, or environmental stimulus that triggers the body to go on high alert "fight-or-flight" state and free up all available energy and resources to escape the perceived threat. Since our bodies prioritize a stress response over all other bodily systems, including the digestive and immune system, a chronic or prolonged stress response can throw all other systems out of balance and lead to degeneration and disease. Simply put, a body in stress cannot heal, so essential oils that support the organs of stress can help the body to rebalance and heal.

Digestion: The body needs food to function. The digestive system breaks down food into essential components to fuel the entire body. Every cell in the body—all the tissues, organs and the bodily functions these cells support—require proper digestion to ensure that the nutrients it needs for optimal brain and body function are properly absorbed and assimilated. Unfortunately, it is not just what you eat, but how you eat that ensures the optimal absorption and assimilation of key nutrients.

Blood Sugar Balance: Blood sugar refers to sugar transported through the bloodstream to supply energy to all the cells in our bodies. It is what gives us energy and what, when out of balance, can lead to weight gain, nutrient deficiencies, and potential diseases like diabetes. If your energy levels or your weight are not where you would like them to be, you might consider oils to support the organs that process blood sugar, including the pancreas, adrenals, and liver.

Detoxification: Detoxification is the body's natural process to rest, repair, and heal. It is how the body cleans house and clears out potential illnesses and disease. This process should occur on a daily basis, but with the toxic overload of modern life, sometimes the organs of detoxification can get overwhelmed and toxins—i.e. any substance that creates irritating and harmful effects in the body—can get reabsorbed or stored in fat cells. Toxins can limit the ability of cells to function. Oils that support the detoxification process include those that support the organs of detoxification, including the liver, gall bladder, lymphatic system, and the skin.

Inflammation: Systemic inflammation often has its roots in gut inflammation, known as intestinal permeability or "leaky gut." When the walls of the intestine become inflamed and porous, undigested food, bacteria, toxins, and other pathogens can enter the bloodstream, provoking an immune response and triggering inflammation throughout the body, including the brain. This systemic inflammation can present as symptoms of pain, autoimmunity, anxiety, or depression. A combination of topically applied essential oils that reduce inflammation and repair the intestinal lining can help to heal systemic inflammation.

How to Use this Book

I formulated my first blend purely by intuition. As I mentioned in the introduction, I had hit rock-bottom, and pharmaceutical drugs weren't helping. Friends dropped off essential oils and told me "these will help you." I asked them how, and they merely responded that I was very smart and highly intuitive and I would figure it out.

The truth is I was in a state of such mental exhaustion that I didn't perform my usual insane amount of research, but instead dove in intuitively, testing to see if any of the oils I received might help support my exhausted adrenals. I was expecting to find one, possibly two. But instead, I was guided to five oils, which I combined to create my first blend, an early version of our ADRENAL™ blend. It worked so well that I mustered the energy to research what I had created. The sheer volume of conflicting information was overwhelming and surprisingly ineffective. When I tried to follow standard suggestions for oils to support different organs, I was unimpressed with the results. The blends I had formulated were far more effective. Realizing their healing potential, I decided to start my company and offer these premade formulations to balance different organ systems.

My intention with this book is to make it as easy as possible for you to determine the best oil for your health priority and to have access to a high-quality essential oils. To that end, the blends I mention in the book are all Vibrant Blue Oils proprietary formulations. That said, I also recognize that many readers may like to blend their own formulations, so I have included all the ingredients of Vibrant Blue Oils proprietary blends in the Appendix. You are welcome to use these oils, or your intuition, to create your own custom blends if that speaks to your heart. If you prefer a ready-made solution sourced with the highest quality organic or wildcrafted ingredients, you are invited to purchase

directly at Vibrant Blue Oils. Go to www.vibrantblueoils.com/
bookbonus to access some exclusive coupons.

How Do I Know What Oils to Start With?

I want to help you support all of the areas where the body can
fall out of balance. The key is to find which particular area is the
most out of balance in your system and start there. Sometimes
the act of supporting the weakest link can help support the entire
system. I have included several quizzes in this book to help you
identify and prioritize your key issues. To help identify your health
priorities, you can also visit www.vibrantblueoils.com/bookbonus
for access to our online self-assessment quiz.

How to Apply Oils—Inhalation

Inhalation is the most effective method of consuming essential
oils as our sense of smell is the most powerful channel into the
body. The easiest way to apply essential oils is literally just to
smell them. Open the bottle, hold it a few inches below your nose,
and inhale deeply. You can also put a drop of oil on your hands,
rub them together, and cup your hands over your nose. Another
inhalation option includes putting a drop or two on a cotton
ball or tissue and placing it in your shirt pocket (or tucking it in
your bra).

Before bed, you can also place a few drops of oil on your
pillowcase or on a cotton ball near your bed to get a mildly diffused
inhalation effect throughout the night. Or you can place a small
bowl of Epsom salt on the night table and add 10 to 15 drops
of essential oils to the salt. The salt slows the evaporation rate
of the oils, so you'll get a longer diffusion throughout the night.

You can also diffuse oils into the air. Diffusing is not as
effective or direct as other inhalation or topical application

methods for balancing different organs or regions of the brain, but it can be highly effective for neutralizing environmental toxins and mold. When choosing a diffuser, cold diffusion using a nebulizer is preferable, as heat can destroy some of the constituents of the oils. If you choose a diffuser that uses heat, ceramic or glass are superior to plastic.

Another alternative to diffusing oils is steam inhalation. Simply pour hot water into a bowl and add two to three drops of your preferred oil. Thoroughly stir the oils into the water, and lean your face over the steaming bowl (you can cover your face with a towel to concentrate the steam) for approximately one minute.

Applying Essential Oils Topically

The combination of the skin's permeability to fat-soluble substances and the small size of essential oil molecules make topical application an ideal channel for balancing different organ systems or stimulating various regions of the brain.

As you may know, the brain needs oxygen, glucose, and stimulation to function. This stimulation can come in the form of stimulatory essential oils. For example, Vibrant Blue Oils PARASYMPATHETIC™ blend can be topically applied behind the ear lobe on the mastoid bone to stimulate the vagal nerve—the on/off switch between the "rest and digest" parasympathetic state of the nervous system and the sympathetic fight-or-flight state.

Applying Oils to the Bottoms of the Feet

All oils can be applied to the bottoms of the feet as the skin there is thicker and less likely to react. The bottoms of the feet contain physical and emotional reflexology points that correspond to the meridians in all of your internal organs, muscular system, skeletal system, and other parts of the body. Because of the correspondences with the internal organs and systems, applying stimulation on the surface of the ear or to the bottoms of the feet can effectively treat the entire body.

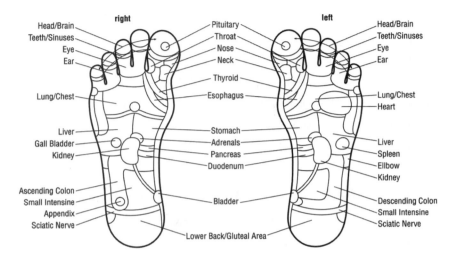

Applying Essential Oils to the Ears

The outermost part of the ear is an ideal application point for emotion balance blends, as it contains emotional reflexology points that correspond to specific emotions and meridians of your internal organs. Applying mild pressure to the reflexology points aids in removing emotional and physical blocks and can help restore balance to the body. This handy chart shows you exactly where to apply to the outer ear for specific emotions.

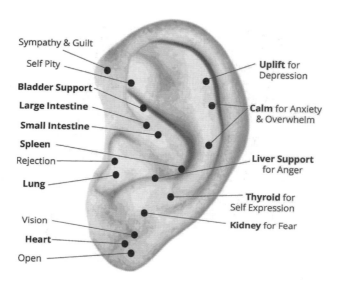

Sympathy & Guilt
Self Pity
Bladder Support
Large Intestine
Small Intestine
Spleen
Rejection
Lung
Vision
Heart
Open

Uplift for Depression
Calm for Anxiety & Overwhelm
Liver Support for Anger
Thyroid for Self Expression
Kidney for Fear

In addition to targeting a specific reflex point, you can rub the entire ear to reduce pain, lower blood pressure, balance hormones, and release endorphins into your system. Your ear lobes are energetically linked to your brain. When the right ear lobe is massaged, it allows the left brain and pituitary gland to become stimulated. When the left ear lobe is massaged it allows the right brain and pineal gland to become stimulated, giving you a whole brain experience. Just use your thumb and index fingers to massage your ear lobes gently in small circles. Rubbing your ears with essential oils a few times a day for as little as a minute is an easy way to return your body to balance.

Applying Essential Oils on the Forehead

The forehead contains several reflex points that can be stimulated with essential oils to help with emotional release. Several practitioners who use essential oils in their practice have shared that these forehead points often deliver more effective results than the organ points or the ears for oil application.

The forehead plays host to several neurovascular points, named "Bennett reflexes," after chiropractor Terrence Bennett who first discovered them in the 1930s.

Stimulation of these points is believed to affect the circulation of the vascular system of various organs and glands to improve many physical and emotional conditions. For example, it is thought to strengthen the connection between the meridians and the nervous system to support the reprogramming of our emotional and mental responses to stress and trauma.

Applying essential oils to or touching these reflex points in three specific areas of the forehead – inside the eyebrows, over the temples, and at the base of the hairline on both the right and left hemisphere of the forehead – can increase cerebral, spinal, organ, and muscle flow of blood to the body. It's hypothesized that when we are under stress, blood goes to the back of the brain where the past is stored. Placing a hand or appropriate essential oils over these points on the forehead helps shift the energy and blood flow from the more emotional mid-brain areas to the area just below the forehead known as the prefrontal cortex, which is associated with a calmer mind and rational, logical thinking.

Emotion-balancing essential oils on the forehead have been shown to calm the vascular system, which circulates the blood flow in the veins, arteries, and heart and further helps alleviate the negative emotions around that issue. Similarly, applying essential oils on specific neurovascular points, while at the same time holding a specific trauma or crisis in the mind, can help the body to release the thought pattern and related stress response that may have become habitual.

The hands can also be used to stimulate the forehead points, but research indicates that the longer you hold the points, the more the stress will fade. Applying essential oils to the points allows you to hold the energy for significantly longer, resulting in greater health improvements.

This technique has been successfully integrated in combination with clinical techniques like Five Element Meridian Release and the Emotional Stress Release taught in "Touch for Health."

Safety Precautions

Be careful never to apply essential oils in the ear canal, near the eyes, or on an open wound. Oils can be easily absorbed through cuts, scrapes, abrasions, burns, and eczema.

Always test a nickel-sized portion on the inside of the arm or another area of skin to make sure your skin can handle the oil before using. In the event of any redness or reaction, apply another oil, like coconut oil or olive oil, over the essential oil application to dilute it. Do not use water, as it might further aggravate the reaction.

Start Slowly

For the first few days of usage, I encourage you to dilute the essential oil with another oil, like coconut or olive oil, and gradually work up to a recommended dosage. Keep in mind that the viscosity of the oil you use will impact how easily the oils penetrate the skin. Sweet almond oil and grape seed oil are less viscous and will penetrate the skin more easily than thicker oils like olive oil, coconut oil, or almond oil.

Applying essential oils to pulse points, like the wrists, the temples, and the back of the neck where the blood vessels are the closest to the skin, also allows for quicker absorption and helps them get to work faster. Absorption can also occur through the hair follicles and sweat ducts. Factors that increase the blood flow to the surface of the skin, such as clean skin and pores, the rate of circulation, and the warmth of the skin, also increase the skin's ability to absorb the oils. Activities that increase circulation and warmth, like hot showers, baths, exercise, massage, saunas, or sitting in a warm room, will increase the rate of absorption.

Less is More

Essential oils are highly concentrated and extremely potent. A drop or two can produce significant results because an entire plant, when distilled, might produce only a single drop of essential oil. They are approximately 75 to 100 times more concentrated, and consequently far more potent, than dried herbs. For example, one drop of peppermint essential oil is considered the therapeutic equivalent to 26 to 28 cups of peppermint tea.

That said, less is often more. Essential oils application may be likened to the use of an eyedropper, not a fire hose. Smelling the bottle a few inches below the nose for three to seven breaths is often sufficient. In fact, at a certain point, you may find you can no longer smell the blend.

This is often an indication that the brain has recognized and transmitted the information of the essential oil molecule. When the sense of smell is satisfied, we often stop detecting the fragrance, as no more is needed at this time. It is a similar mechanism to how we stop eating when our sense of hunger has been satisfied.

Essential oils are very powerful tools for naturally shifting the body into balance and can trigger both a physical or emotional detoxifying response, especially when applied too aggressively. In fact, research has proven that desired effects of essential oils are drastically minimized or even negated when more than a faint scent was detectable. When the air inhaled had a noticeable aroma, the effectiveness of the oils actually decreased.

For that reason, I recommend starting very gradually, first smelling the oil for a few days, then diluting heavily with each topical application to gradually work up to a full dosage. This gradual introduction reduces the chances of an intense reaction.

Even when the emotions are released slowly and gradually, it can be overwhelming. I equate the experience to cleaning out a storage place in our house. It often gets messier before it gets cleaner. We have to pull everything out of our neatly tucked away hiding spaces, look at it and decide what needs to be tossed, kept, or further processed. The same is true for our emotions. Some emotions no longer serve and are relatively easy to discard, while others require additional processing before we are ready to let them go.

On that note, a few drops are more than enough for any application. Like homeopathy, essential oils can be more effective in low amounts. When diffusing, only use the oil to the level of detection (being able to smell it) for short intervals, no more than 20 minutes at a time.

Trust your Sense of Smell

We are intuitively drawn to what our body needs, both in our sense of smell and our sense of taste. For example, you may crave a hamburger if you need iron or chocolate if you need magnesium. It's important to trust your intuition and your sense of smell, as it will often guide you to what your body needs.

I have observed both personally and with clients that the oils seem to change their fragrance when the body needs them. One client reported that "the **INTESTINAL MUCOSA**™ always smells the best to me, so divine that I just want to eat it up—which makes sense, because my small intestine suffered the most damage with my ulcerative colitis. When I first began using the **GALLBLADDER**™, I reacted to it in the same way—I couldn't get enough of it and I kept craving the fragrance. After my gallbladder started to heal, I suddenly stopped craving it and didn't find the smell as enticing."

Trust that when you crave a fragrance, it is your body's innate intelligence communicating what it needs to be healthy. This does not necessarily mean that an oil will not be beneficial to you if you don't enjoy the fragrance, but you may find yourself inexplicably drawn to a particular oil because your body is asking for it.

How often to use them?

I recommend you use essential oils a minimum of twice daily. If it is hard to remember to use them, just keep them by your toothbrush and apply when you first wake up and before bed. As you notice that the blends help you, you can carry them in your purse or pocket and apply as often as every 20 minutes.

How to use them?

I recommend smelling them or applying topically, either over a particular organ, on the bottoms of the feet or the outside of the ears (never in the ear canal). You can find specific application points along with directions to help you apply them at www.vibrantblueoils.com/bookbonus, but I also encourage you to use your intuition. For additional resources to help you get started with essential oils, go to www.vibrantblueoils.com/bookbonus.

Using more than one blend at once?

I am often asked if it is ok to use more than one blend at the same time. The short answer is Yes! Layering oil blends can actually have a synergistic effect, enhancing and optimizing the effectiveness of the combined oils. This is one of the reasons we have created kits of three oil blends designed to be used in combination with each other, including the **STRESS SUPPORT KIT, BLOOD SUGAR SUPPORT KIT, GUT REPAIR KIT, DETOX SUPPORT KIT, DIGESTION SUPPORT** and **BRAIN SUPPORT KIT**. In addition, our **PARASYMPATHETIC**™

blend consistently seems to enhance all other blends when used in combination. Similarly, the **ANTI-INFLAMMATORY**™ blend can be combined with any Body Balance blend to reduce organ specific inflammation. That said, I do not recommend applying more than three blends at any given time of application. Applying too many oils at the same time can be overwhelming and confusing to the body.

How will I know if it is working?

You will know the oil is working when you begin to feel better. One of my best customers, Andrea, wrote to tell me how grateful she was when our oils brought her out of a dark period of constant pain, fatigue, and brain fog that limited her ability to work, travel, and enjoy her children. If you are in this state and an oil helps you, you will carry that oil with you everywhere. As you begin to heal, you may notice that you need the oil less and less. You may become less anxious or worried, able to sleep through the night, or enjoy a meal and not feel sick after.

The wonderful thing about healing is that once we feel better, we often forget how awful we felt before. When we start to feel better, most of us forget that we once suffered from pain, fatigue, or brain fog.

Questions?

Join our Vibrant Blue Oils Facebook Discussion Group to get your personal questions answered. You can find the link at www.vibrantblueoils.com/bookbonus.

Chapter 3

The Parasympathetic State

The body has a natural balance and rhythm: the sleep and wake cycles, the digestion and elimination cycles, and the cycle in which the body responds to stress and returns to the balanced parasympathetic state to rest, digest, and heal.

As long as we maintain this delicate balance, called homeostasis, we feel healthy. When we fall out of balance for too long, our health begins to decline. The key to this balance is the ability to return to the parasympathetic state where the body can rest, digest, and heal after a stress response passes.

What Is the Parasympathetic State?

The parasympathetic state is one of the two divisions of the autonomic nervous system, which regulates the body's unconscious actions, like digestion, immunity, adrenal function, cardiovascular health, brain health, and detoxification.

It is the counterpart to the sympathetic "fight-or-flight" state, which is the body's first line of defense against stress. In the sympathetic state, the body kicks into survival mode. It releases hormones, like adrenaline, which make the heart beat faster. Blood pressure and breathing increase to help transport nutrients and oxygen to the cells faster, the pupils dilate so we can see more clearly, and the blood pumps to external muscles so we can flee faster. The blood flows away from internal organs of digestion, which turns off the digestive process.

It also shuts down all functions that are not necessary to survival, like the immune system, inflammation, reproduction, and rational thinking. This can be a helpful tip to know if you are trying to communicate with someone and it isn't going well. Look to see if their pupils are dilated (black parts enlarged). It's a clue that they are locked in that sympathetic state and will not be able to engage in a rational way.

We are designed to drop into this sympathetic "fight-or-flight" state and flee from danger, then return to the parasympathetic state, which brings the body back to normal, relaxed functioning. Muscles relax, the mind slows down, and digestion increases. The body concentrates on digesting and absorbing nutrients and on building reserves for future emergencies.

The parasympathetic state is the realm of deep rest and relaxation; it is a necessary state for our bodies to digest, detoxify, support immune function, regenerate and. heal. Unfortunately, many of us get stuck in the sympathetic state, denying our bodies the opportunity to properly rebuild and recover.

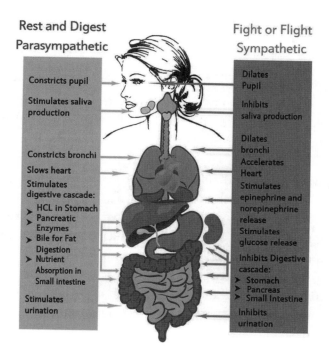

Rest and Digest
Parasympathetic

Fight or Flight
Sympathetic

Constricts pupil

Stimulates saliva production

Constricts bronchi

Slows heart

Stimulates digestive cascade:
➤ HCL in Stomach
➤ Pancreatic Enzymes
➤ Bile for Fat Digestion
➤ Nutrient Absorption in Small intestine

Stimulates urination

Dilates Pupil

Inhibits saliva production

Dilates bronchi

Accelerates Heart

Stimulates epinephrine and norepinephrine release

Stimulates glucose release

Inhibits Digestive cascade:
➤ Stomach
➤ Pancreas
➤ Small Intestine

Inhibits urination

Symptoms of the Sympathetic State

- ❏ Dry mouth
- ❏ Acid indigestion (GERD)
- ❏ SIBO
- ❏ Bloating
- ❏ Constipation
- ❏ Detoxification challenges, including Gall Bladder pain
- ❏ Chronic infections
- ❏ Blood Sugar Dysregulation

How Do We Get Stuck in the Sympathetic State?

Our nervous systems were designed to respond to short and acute stress responses, like the experience of running from a

51

predator. When the cause of the stress is removed, the body is designed to drop back into the parasympathetic state and return to normal function.

Unfortunately, most of the modern day stress we experience from school, our jobs, our relationships, traffic, or even watching the news or a scary movie never goes away. This chronic and prolonged stress forces the body to provide longer-term protection against the stress, often recruiting other organs like the hypothalamus and the adrenals to contribute to the stress response (more about this in Chapter 5).

It is also important to understand that a stressor is defined as anything that can knock us out of balance. Stress can be physical, environmental, physiological, or even emotional. In fact, the body cannot differentiate between actual physical stress and emotional or anticipatory stress, like thinking about a catastrophe that might occur in some imaginary future or reliving a traumatic experience from the past.

The book, *Why Zebras Don't Get Ulcers*, talks about this phenomenon, noting "sometimes we are smart enough to see things coming and, based only on anticipation, turn on a stress-response as robust as if the event had actually occurred."

This is an important point to land on because most of us assume that our stress is related to external stresses like challenging relationships, traffic, deadlines, or financial pressures.

In truth, internal stressors from thought patterns related to emotions like fear, worry, anger, grief, resentment, recalling past trauma, or even excessive ambition and perfectionism, trigger the sympathetic state. Grief, in particular, can tax the body. This is one of the reasons that people so often die shortly after the passing of a partner.

When we incur this chronic and prolonged stress, with no down time to rest and recover between stress responses, we stay locked in the chronic sympathetic state, known as sympathetic dominance.

Unfortunately, our bodies were not built to withstand these effects of chronic and prolonged stress. When we get stuck in the sympathetic fight or flight mode, our bodies can't reboot and heal. Even racecars need to make pit stops along the way to prevent their tires from blowing out. But so many of us forget to make those pit stops, those small pauses that allow our bodies to rest and repair.

After a stress response, the body can reach a resolution that turns off the sympathetic system and drops back into the parasympathetic. But sometimes, when the stressful situation is ongoing (or perceived as such), or we push too hard or worry too much without enough downtime for recovery between stress responses, our bodies can stay locked in the sympathetic nervous system "fight-or-flight" response.

Kind of like never turning off the light, our sympathetic system gets stuck in that "on" position, which keeps our parasympathetic "rest and digest" response stuck in the "off" position.

This is an important point to understand. Your body needs to exit out of the sympathetic mode to be able to enter into the parasympathetic mode. When it is stuck in sympathetic, it never gets to drop into that parasympathetic state that is critical for allowing the body to rest, repair, and heal.

If this adaptation response continues for a prolonged time without periods of relaxation and rest, the result is fatigue, concentration lapses, irritability, and lethargy as the effort to sustain arousal slides into negative stress.

What is Sympathetic Dominance?

Sympathetic dominance is a term coined by Dr. Lawrence Wilson that indicates a pattern of over-utilizing the sympathetic nervous system either by pushing too hard or worrying too much without time to reset and return to homeostasis. Sympathetic dominance often occurs when there is not enough downtime for recovery between stress responses.

Sympathetic-dominant individuals tend to be smart and have very active minds, which easily become overactive. They may have had an upbringing in which they were taught not to be lazy, to be productive, to not waste time. This influence can lead them to become compulsive or obsessive, or they may experience emotions of fear, anger, worry, and other negative feelings that drive them to high achievement or just to keep moving all the time. This can make relaxing, sleeping, or just sitting even more difficult because the body is often in a "second wind" mode of living much of the time.

Sympathetic System

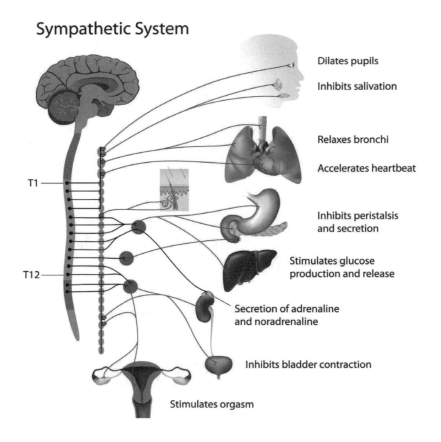

T1

T12

Dilates pupils

Inhibits salivation

Relaxes bronchi

Accelerates heartbeat

Inhibits peristalsis and secretion

Stimulates glucose production and release

Secretion of adrenaline and noradrenaline

Inhibits bladder contraction

Stimulates orgasm

Sympathetic-Dominant Personality Type

- ☐ Patterns of extreme physical activity
- ☐ Forever busy
- ☐ Difficulty relaxing, sitting still, resting, and being idle
- ☐ Highly driven and compelled
- ☐ Somewhat obsessive or compulsive
- ☐ Often stressed as if being "chased by tigers"
- ☐ Belief that to relax is a "waste of time" or "unproductive" or "lazy"
- ☐ Identification as a "doer" with lots of physical or mental activities
- ☐ Struggling to be happy without needing to run around or do much of anything
- ☐ Anxious or worriers. This is a form of "running around aimlessly" in the mind
- ☐ Tired, but usually somewhat out of touch with the fatigue and exhaustion
- ☐ Feeling tired only when you slow down. If you relax, you feel like going to sleep
- ☐ A very active or analytical mind
- ☐ Willful, often willing themselves to think and do too much
- ☐ Fearful and always somewhat depressed underneath due to fears, worries, and fatigue
- ☐ Constant activity or busyness to avoid feeling these unpleasant emotions
- ☐ Desire to "move on," but unsure how to do this
- ☐ Somewhat lonely while trying to "fit in with the crowd"
- ☐ Overworked, overachiever, and generally run ragged
- ☐ Tries to please others and exhausts self in the process
- ☐ Ungrounded and not centered enough. This goes with the tendency to run around too much or worry too much

The Body Locked in the Sympathetic State?

Because the body needn't bother with digestion in the midst of a life-threatening crisis, blood vessels traveling to the gastrointestinal system constrict, shunting blood preferentially to the large muscle groups in the extremities, including the heart and the brain, allowing the heart to pump harder, the thighs to run faster, the brain to process more quickly, and the pupils to dilate so you can see more clearly to spot an attacker and find your escape route.

Your body cannot optimally digest, absorb, and assimilate nutrients when you are locked in the sympathetic state. The brain and the autonomic nervous system need to be in a parasympathetic state to trigger all the parasympathetic responses in the digestive cascade, including:

> - **Mouth** to trigger the production and release of saliva, which helps break down and digest our food.
> - **Stomach** to produce and release stomach acid, for optimal digestion. Stomach acid, in particular, helps us digest our proteins more completely. The parasympathetic state also triggers the sphincter between the stomach and esophagus to close, preventing acid reflux from stomach to esophagus.
> - **Pancreas** to release enzymes for digestion to efficiently digest all the protein, carbs, and fats you are consuming in your diet.
> - **Gallbladder** to release bile for fat digestion in the duodenum and detoxification of old hormones. Bile acids are mainly toxic metabolites and waste products from the liver; so improved bile flow also improves detoxification.
> - **Liver** to support detoxification and blood sugar functions.
> - **Small Intestine** to receive increased blood flow, allowing for healing of the intestinal wall and optimal enzymatic

activity and nutrient assimilation. The parasympathetic state also activates the beneficial effects of the probiotic bacteria in the gut and triggers peristalsis, the muscle contractions that move food and waste through the digestive tract, known as the "Housekeeping Wave". A lack of motility can lead to dysbiosis (a microbial imbalance), including small intestine bacterial overgrowth (SIBO).

> **Large Intestine**—to eliminate waste. Inducing the parasympathetic state triggers peristalsis, the muscle contractions of the intestines that move the stool, making this a great solution for constipation issues.

When the body is locked in the sympathetic state, it continues to release stress hormones. It's like they are stuck in the "on" position, too!

The brain triggers the adrenal glands to release hormones like cortisol that help us access instant energy. Cortisol also turns off any systems that can get in the way of a rapid response. For example, cortisol suppresses the immune system to reduce the inflammatory response that might accompany an attack that a life-or-death situation might inflict on your body. Cortisol effectively turns off inflammation, which is one of the reasons that the similar medication cortisone is used to reduce inflammation.

When locked in the sympathetic state, the body also stops all routine maintenance, shutting off its natural self-repair mechanisms, like those that fight infection, prevent cancer, repair broken proteins, and fend off disease. There's no point in wasting all the body's precious energy preventing disease or healing from an illness if you're about to die anyway, right?

The immune system also disengages, as it is aligned with the inflammatory response and therefore suppressed by the stress response. A diminished immune response has implications on all levels, from vulnerability to infections to a lack of protection from viruses, autoimmunity, or even cancer.

While a reduction in such functions makes sense during a life-threatening emergency, it is not a good thing to get stuck permanently in that mode. Right?

Inflammation is the body's attempt at self-protection. It causes tissues to swell up, creates heat, and causes nearby muscles to contract to isolate whatever is happening in that area, so it doesn't spread throughout the body.

The immune system plays a similar role, isolating and attacking any foreign or harmful substances to protect the body. When these two defense mechanisms are turned off for extended periods of time, it can deplete our reserves of nutrients and hormones, much like deficit spending. At a certain point, this can catch up to you, leaving you vulnerable to health issues like depression or, in some cases, heart disease, auto immunity, and even cancer.

But there is a solution. You can manually override the parasympathetic response.

How to Trigger the Parasympathetic State

When your phone or computer malfunctions, often you can restart it, and it seems to work perfectly. (Which is a good thing because it is my one and only technology hack!) Don't you wish it could be that easy with our bodies? What if we could just reboot our systems and reset our stress levels? Well, it actually kind of is.

There are techniques for hacking the parasympathetic state. That's right. Just like you can reboot your computer or your phone, you can reboot your body by manually overriding the on/off switch between the sympathetic "fight-or-flight" state and the parasympathetic "rest-and-digest" state of the nervous system.

Yes. You heard me correctly. The body has a reboot button, just like your phone. And it's located at the vagus nerve, cranial nerve #10. That's vagus, V-A-G-U-S, not the city in Nevada that is known for its showgirls and gambling, but similarly exciting regarding the upside it presents.

Stimulating the vagus nerve where the nerve endings are most accessible to the surface of the skin is a key to triggering the body's "rest-and-digest" parasympathetic nervous system response.

Essential Oils for the Parasympathetic State

To stimulate the parasympathetic nervous system, apply 1–2 drops of **PARASYMPATHETIC**™, or another stimulatory oil, on the vagus nerve (behind the ear, anterior to the mastoid bone on the neck). This stimulates the nerve endings in the skin, which then triggers the parasympathetic nervous system response. Use it before meals or during times of intense stress. It can also be applied to the base of the skull or smelled.

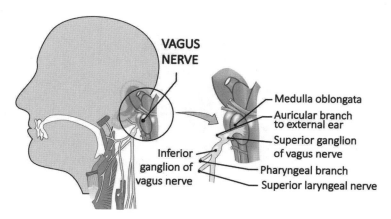

What is the Vagus Nerve?

The vagus nerve is the key to triggering the parasympathetic state. It is one of two extremely long cranial nerves that start at the base of the brain and travel down the neck on both sides of the body near the carotid artery and jugular vein, across the chest and down through the abdomen, triggering the parasympathetic response in every organ of digestion.

Organs Connected to the Vagus Nerve

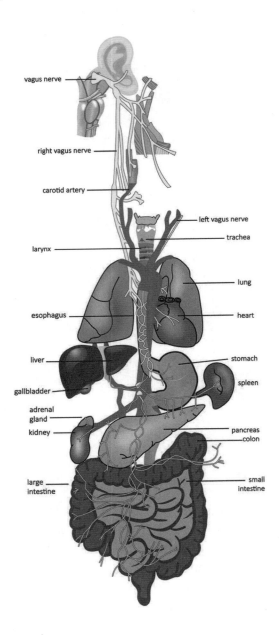

The vagus nerve, the longest nerve in the body, delivers bi-directional signals between the brain and the body. This means it sends signals from the brain to activate various organs and it delivers information from the organs back to the brain. We can say it serves as the master controller of immune cells, organs, and stem cells, along with mood, digestion, memory, cognitive function, and blood pressure. You can see that it impacts many aspects of health.

"Vagus" is Latin for "wandering." As the name implies, the vagus nerve travels through the body, networking the brain with the stomach and digestive system; visceral organs, including the lungs, heart, spleen, intestines, liver and kidneys; and a range of other nerves that are involved in speech, eye contact, facial expressions, and even your ability to tune into other people's voices.

It is made of thousands and thousands of fibers, and 80 percent of them are sensory, meaning that the vagus nerve reports back to your brain the activity in your organs. Some people have stronger vagus tone, which means their bodies can relax faster after stress. Low vagus tone has been associated with chronic inflammation and other health concerns.

For example, issues with dental amalgams and heavy-metal-triggered autism may be linked to poor vagus signaling. The heavy metal mercury is a known neurotoxin that blocks the action of acetylcholine, the neurotransmitter used by the vagus nerve to signal the heart muscle. The immune system attempts to neutralize mercury from dental amalgam fillings in the mouth or from vaccinations that cross the blood brain barrier via lymph nodes. Because lymph nodes run along the sides of the neck, near the vagus nerve, the mercury can impact the vagus nerve and its ability to signal the body.

In *The Polyvagal Theory: Neurophysiological Foundations of Emotions, Attachment, Communication, and Self-regulation*, Dr. Stephen Porges identifies how the frequently observed rocking and swinging behaviors in autistic individuals may reflect a naturally occurring bio-behavioral strategy to stimulate and regulate a vagal system that is not functioning efficiently.

Improving Vagal Tone and Function

Neurologists in the nineteenth century realized that applying pressure on the carotid artery in the neck (i.e. the vagus nerve) could stop seizures. This prompted significant research trials to manually stimulate the vagus nerve with electrical impulses sent through a device that is surgically implanted under the skin of the chest, similar to a pacemaker. When activated, the device sends electrical signals along the vagus nerve to the brainstem, which then sends signals to certain areas in your brain.

Vagus nerve stimulation has been used to treat epilepsy, depression, multiple sclerosis, migraines, and Alzheimer's disease. The Food and Drug Administration has officially approved vagus nerve stimulation for epilepsy and depression.

While the benefits of this surgical procedure are exciting, the potential to stimulate the vagus nerve through the non-invasive methods are equally compelling.

There are several ways to stimulate the vagus nerve, including mindful breathing, gargling, using a tongue depressor to stimulate a gag reflex, or applying extremely cold water to the face or neck.

Like surgery, these techniques are a little intense for me, so instead, I prefer to apply a stimulatory blend of essential oils to the point where the vagus nerve is most accessible to the surface of the skin: behind the earlobe and up one inch (on either side of the neck) on the mastoid bone.

The skin is relatively permeable to small molecules of fat-soluble substances like essential oils. This means stimulatory essential oils are easily absorbed through the skin and can be used much like an electrical impulse to trigger the parasympathetic nervous system's rest-and-digest response.

Shifting back into the parasympathetic state allows healing and regeneration to occur. It was by far the most powerful tool I used in my recovery from depression.

It is also an easy and convenient hack to reset your body so you can perform parasympathetic activities like digesting, detoxifying, lowering blood pressure, and building immunity. It's great to practice before meals, as it turns on your body's ability to digest, absorb, and assimilate your nutrients.

How You Might Feel in Parasympathetic State

You can hear direct evidence that parasympathetic stimulation is happening: your tummy will rumble increasingly as you relax. The person who has been on a stressful adrenaline habit for years will probably feel tired and ill once beginning to relax. They are feeling the true state of affairs in the body rather than the false energy from being on adrenaline. As the healing progresses and the reserves are built up again, this will pass.

Benefits of the Parasympathetic State

Digestion only occurs when we are in the parasympathetic state of our nervous system. It is the "rest-and-digest" mode of the body. When we enter the parasympathetic mode, it triggers the digestive cascade. When you stimulate the parasympathetic nervous system, all downstream digestive function improves. By triggering the shift into parasympathetic mode, PARASYMPATHETIC™ uniquely optimizes digestion, absorption, and assimilation.

Not only will you correct any short-term problems, but you will reset the stress response by building vagus tone. This can improve all aspects of health related to the vagus nerve triggering the parasympathetic state.

Vagus Nerve and Heart Health

Our heart rate is controlled by the two branches of the autonomic nervous system (ANS). The "fight or flight" sympathetic nervous system raises our heart rate so we can pump more blood to our muscles and flee from danger, while the "rest and digest" parasympathetic nervous system slows down our heart rate so we can rest, repair and recover.

The delicate balance between the two states of the autonomic nervous system is known as homeostasis. The vagus nerve, which originates in the brain and wraps around our heart and organs of digestion, controls this delicate balance, serving as a temperature gauge over the body's relaxation response, including the heart rate.

The vagus nerve acts as the "reset" button, communicating bi-directional signals to the body and brain that the danger has passed and it is safe to return to the relaxed parasympathetic state.

In the parasympathetic state, the vagus nerve releases the neurotransmitter acetylcholine to the sinoatrial node of the heart signaling it to prolong the time to the next heartbeat, thus slowing the pulse. This slowing of successive heartbeats is known as heart rate variability (HRV).

HRV is often used as both an index of sympathetic to parasympathetic balance of heart rate fluctuation as well as a predictive measure of health and mortality. In fact, HRV data indicates that decreased vagus nerve activity is often associated with increased morbidity and mortality from cardiac surgery or myocardial infarction along with other health concerns.

The Vagus Nerve and Inflammation

The vagus nerve also plays a key role in reducing systemic inflammation which can contribute to heart problems. The vagus nerve communicates with the rest of the body by releasing the neurotransmitter acetylcholine.

Stimulating the vagus nerve sends acetylcholine throughout the body, not only making us feel relaxed, but also acting as a brake on inflammation in the body. This may be why supplementing with acetylcholine can have many of the same effects as vagal stimulation because this is how the vagus nerve stimulates various organs.

Termed 'the inflammatory reflex', the vagus nerve senses peripheral inflammation and sends a message to the spleen (which is responsible for a lot of immune system regulation) to inhibit the production of pro-inflammatory cytokines.

Without the influence of the vagus nerve releasing acetylcholine, cytokines may be produced in much larger quantities in response to stimuli that would have been otherwise harmless in the presence of a functioning neural circuit.

This is great news for heart health, as inflammation accelerates the progression of heart disease, contributing to of atherosclerotic plaque deposits and leading to myocardial and cerebral infarction.

In addition, cardiovascular disease can be triggered by the action of cytokine produced C-reactive protein (CRP). Several studies have shown an inverse relationship between HRV and CRP levels.

As previously mentioned, the ability of the vagus nerve to send signals to the body can be compromised from chronic stress and toxins like heavy metals. Fortunately, essential oils can play a critical role in improving the ability of the vagus nerve to send and receive signals.

Other Benefits of Vagus Nerve Stimulation

Lowers blood pressure. Vagus nerve stimulation has been shown to decrease blood pressure, heart rate, and breathing rate. Healthy blood pressure depends on healthy vagus nerve tone. When stimulated correctly, the nerve will dramatically lower blood pressure in a very short period, with no side effects.

Reduces depression. Stimulating the vagus nerve has proven to be extremely effective in treating non-responsive depression. The vagus nerve releases the neurotransmitter acetylcholine, which is responsible for memory and learning, and signals the body to relax and calm down. "Stimulating the vagus nerve sends acetylcholine throughout the body, not only relaxing you, but also turning down the fires of inflammation (and regulating the immune system)," writes Dr. Mark Hyman in *The UltraMind Solution*.

Improves cognitive function. Studies reveal increased attention and memory performance from epileptic patients who stimulated their vagus nerve, in part because the main relay station for the vagus nerve projects into areas of the brain involved in learning and memory formation (amygdala, hippocampus).

Decreases migraines. In a recent study, scientists demonstrated that stimulation of the vagus nerve reduced the frequency of migraine headaches by over 50 percent, as well as a marked reduction in epileptic seizures.

Chapter 4

Sleep

Restful sleep, defined as the ability to fall asleep and stay asleep for seven to eight hours per night, is the cornerstone of health, impacting both its quality and your ability to heal. It is during restful sleep that the body rests, regenerates, repairs, detoxifies, balances blood sugar levels, burns calories, supports immune activity, and resets our energy reserves..

Sleep is critical for basic maintenance and repair of the neurological, endocrine, immune, musculoskeletal, and digestive systems. Restful sleep can:

➤ Elevate mental clarity and memory
➤ Enhance athletic performance
➤ Boosts mood and energy
➤ Improve immune function
➤ Increase our tolerance to stress

Without restful sleep, we feel fatigued, and our body compensates with cortisol spikes, sugar cravings, and other tricks to keep us awake and functioning. Unfortunately, it is not enough to consume a nutrient dense diet with appropriate supplements. If you are not sleeping well, it will be much harder to heal.

Poor Sleep is an Epidemic

Many people, including small children, suffer from some sleep dysfunction. Many of us either have trouble falling asleep or staying asleep, resulting in fewer than six hours of sleep per night, which is often associated with low-grade chronic inflammation.

This inadequate rest can impair our ability to think, to handle stress, to maintain a healthy immune system, and to moderate our emotions. Poor sleep is also correlated with heart disease, hypertension, weight gain, diabetes, and a wide range of psychiatric disorders including depression and anxiety.

Poor Sleep Impacts Your Health

Research shows that poor sleep—less than 6 hours per night—significantly increases the risk of poor health conditions, including diabetes, obesity, cardiovascular disease, cancer, and autoimmune disease.

In her book *Go to Bed*, Paleo Mom Sarah Ballantyne finds that:

➤ Sleep disorders increase the risk of developing an autoimmune condition by 50 percent.
➤ Sleeping less than 6 hours per night increases the risk of obesity by 55 percent in adults (90 percent in children!).
➤ Sleeping less than 6 hours per night increases the risk of type 2 diabetes by 50 percent.
➤ Routinely sleeping less than six hours per night doubles the risk of stroke, doubles the risk of myocardial infarction, increases the risk of congestive heart failure by 67 percent, and increases the risk of coronary heart disease by 48 percent.

> ➤ The amount of sleep you get upon and after breast cancer diagnosis is a predictor of survival, and getting less than six hours of sleep increases the risk of death by 46 percent.

This correlation with disease can be attributed to how sleep throws off other cycles in the body.

Sleep Cycles Impact Other Cycles

There is growing evidence that sleep cycles impact other cycles in the body, including the rhythmic patterns of the digestive and immune systems. When we sleep, the brain produces 90-minute cycles of slow wave sleep. Periods of rapid eye movement (REM) follow, during which time dreams occur. During the night, the gut also produces 90-minute slow wave muscle contractions, followed by short bursts of rapid movement. Poor sleep cycles can disrupt this digestive function and the healing process within the gut.

Low Melatonin Can Impact Gut Health

The sleep cycle, beginning with the release of the hormone melatonin from the pineal gland, appears to support the body's immune system by resetting the balance of healthy bacteria in the small intestine. Melatonin, in combination with the hormone prolactin, triggers an immune response that regenerates the microflora and epithelial lining in the small intestine to restore a healthy balance and negate the threat of viruses, bacteria, and other toxins in the body.

Eight hours of sleep is optimal for this melatonin and prolactin production to occur. Anything less does not allow these hormones to effectively balance the gut flora, which is key to supporting the immune system. Melatonin is also thought to help regulate inflammation and support glutathione levels.

Balancing Sleep can Balance Adrenal Rhythms

As you may know, the stress hormone cortisol is produced by the adrenal glands. The sleep hormone melatonin is released by the pineal gland, a small pinecone-shaped endocrine gland located near the center of the brain.

Our cortisol rhythms are supposed to be highest in the morning and then wane as the day wears on. When people are active at night and slow in the morning, the cortisol patterns are reversed. This throws off the circadian rhythm and can lead to sleep disruptions, which, in turn, can further impair adrenal function.

This triggers a vicious cycle. Without proper melatonin production from the pineal gland, adrenals will overwork at night. Melatonin needs to help drive down cortisol. When the adrenal hormone cortisol is too high at night, the pineal excretion of melatonin will be inhibited, causing cortisol levels to remain too high, which requires the adrenals to overwork. These high cortisol levels during sleep prevent you from dropping into the appropriate level of REM sleep that allows the body to regenerate, detoxify, and support immune activity. Lack of REM sleep reduces mental vitality and vigor and induces depression. Conversely, if the pineal secretion is excessive in the morning, it's going to depress the output of cortisol, and you won't feel like you've had any rest.

The cortisol rhythms are controlled by the hypothalamus-pituitary-adrenal axis (HPA axis) communication between the hypothalamus, pituitary and adrenal glands, which triggers the adrenals to release cortisol in response to stress. The HPA axis stops releasing cortisol when the negative feedback loop triggers the hypothalamus that there is enough cortisol in the system. Any

HPA dysregulation can throw cortisol rhythms out of balance and with it, the circadian rhythms of the body.

If you treat sleep issues only on the adrenal level by taking adrenal support, you often will not see much improvement. It's important to consider not only how much cortisol the adrenals are producing, but also to look at the cortisol rhythms. Just taking an adrenal supplement to re-balance adrenals may be insufficient. You need to support the limbic system, including the hypothalamus and pineal gland, to reset these rhythms.

Impaired Adrenal Rhythm Impacts:

➤ **Energy Production:** Abnormal adrenal function can alter the ability of cells to produce energy.

➤ **Muscle and Joint Function:** Abnormal adrenal rhythms compromise tissue repair and increase tissue breakdown, leading to muscle and joint pain.

➤ **Bone Health:** The adrenal rhythm determines how well we build bone. If the night and morning cortisol levels are elevated, our bones do not rebuild well.

➤ **Immune Health:** The immune system cycle follows the cortisol cycle. If the cycle is disrupted, especially at night, the immune response in the lungs, throat, urinary tract, and intestines is suppressed.

➤ **Sleep Quality:** The ability to enter REM sleep cycles and experience regenerative sleep is interrupted by high cortisol values at night and in the morning. Chronic lack of REM sleep can reduce a person's mental vitality and vigor and induce depression.

➤ **Skin Regeneration:** Skin regenerates during the night. With higher night cortisol values, less skin regeneration takes place.

> **Thyroid Function**: The level of cortisol at the cell level controls thyroid hormone production. Often, hypothyroid symptoms such as fatigue and low body temperature are due to an adrenal maladaptation.

> **Chronic Fatigue Syndrome**: A common HPA axis defect in CFS is impaired corticotrophin release.

> **Glycemic Dysregulation:** Chronic hypoglycemia can impair normal adrenal function by constant overstimulation of cortisol production. Recurring exposure to high cortisol will impair insulin activity and invariably lead to insulin resistance or diabetes.

> **Allergies/Autoimmune Disorders:** Patients with environmentally triggered allergies and autoimmune diseases dramatically benefited when given cortisol for other purposes. Apparently, the disruption of the adrenal axis and cytokine relationships leads to predisposition and aggravation of autoimmune diseases.

> **Depression:** Several recent publications report a hyperactive HPA axis in depressed patients. Elevated midnight salivary cortisol is now considered one of the best tests in diagnosing endogenous depression. Other anomalies in cortisol rhythm usually accompany the midnight elevation.

> **ADD** Cortisol elevations and rhythm disruptions throughout the day are typical of attention deficit disorders.

How to Solve Sleep Challenges

To solve sleep challenges, you need to look at the underlying issues. These can range from low levels of melatonin in the system, which can make it challenging to fall asleep, to blood sugar and hormonal challenges or an overload of the detoxification organs, such as the liver and gall bladder, which can contribute to nighttime waking.

In searching for an alternative to over-the-counter medications and prescription drugs, I found that sleep issues lend themselves especially well to essential oil support. I have attempted to isolate different sleep issues. At Vibrant Blue Oils (www.vibrantblueoils.com/bookbonus), I have created an online sleep assessment to help you learn more about those specific sleep issues and the natural remedies to consider in place of drugs.

Difficulty Falling Asleep

If you struggle to fall asleep or experience racing thoughts or worries while lying in bed, it can indicate that the body's natural sleep and wake cycles, known as the circadian rhythms, might be a little out of balance.

Cortisol and melatonin have an antagonistic relationship. Elevated cortisol levels at night turn off melatonin production. Similarly, if melatonin is elevated, then cortisol is depressed, throwing off the circadian rhythm.

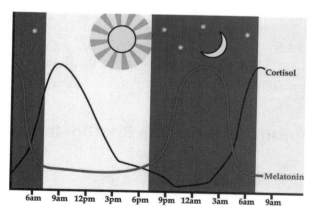

It might help to think of a teeter-totter. When the stress hormone (cortisol) is high, it forces the sleep hormone (melatonin)

to be low. People often supplement with the melatonin hormone, which can help in the short term. The challenge here is that the body, specifically the pineal gland, is supposed to make melatonin, and external supplementation of the hormone sends the signal to the body that it is sufficient in melatonin production. It reduces the body's production of the hormone. In other words, it throws off the body's internal sensor for self-regulation.

Another option is to help the pineal gland return to its innate intelligence and release more melatonin naturally, which we are doing by applying Vibrant Blue Oils **CIRCADIAN RHYTHM™** blend to specific locations on the head (top of the skull, back of the head and on the skull right above the ears). This method emulates the innate intelligence of the body and has been extremely effective for those suffering from sleep issues and anxiety.

If you again think of the teeter-totter example, when melatonin increases, it forces cortisol levels down, effectively serving as a backdoor to lowering stress, anxiety, and the racing thoughts that keep many of us wide awake when our bodies are exhausted and longing for sleep. My 10-year-old daughter suffered from nighttime anxiety for over a year. I tried everything I could think of and often just spent the night holding her while she cried, trying to soothe her fears. The **CIRCADIAN RHYTHM™** blend was a game changer for us. Not only did it help her fall asleep almost instantly, but within a week she reported that her nighttime anxiety was gone.

Symptoms of Circadian Rhythm Imbalance

- ❑ Difficulty falling asleep
- ❑ Tendency to be a "night person"
- ❑ Tendency to be keyed up, trouble calming down
- ❑ Clenching or grinding teeth
- ❑ Difficulty waking up in the morning

- ❑ Inability to feel well rested after sleep
- ❑ Energy drop between 4:00 and 7:00 in the afternoon
- ❑ Increased sleepiness in the winter, especially as the light diminishes
- ❑ Inability to remember dreams
- ❑ Waking up wide awake

Essential Oils for Falling Asleep

The following essential oil blends may be helpful if you struggle to fall asleep:

CIRCADIAN RHYTHM™ blend works well for people who struggle to fall asleep at night because of high stress or racing thoughts. Restful sleep is a critical component to healing. When the circadian rhythms flow smoothly, the body heals more easily. This blend naturally triggers the pineal gland to release melatonin.

The pineal gland is located behind the hypothalamus in the brain. It helps to regulate our body's biological body clock rhythms, known as the circadian rhythms, by producing melatonin in response to changes in light. The pineal gland serves as part of our visual system, receiving signals of changes in natural light from the eyes. Melatonin is, in effect, a "darkness" hormone, because it is made at night. The length of the night influences the duration of melatonin secretion.

To help reset the pineal gland and re-establish healthy circadian rhythms, apply on the very top of the head, the back of the head, and on the skin above the ears. It's ideal to use it in a low-light atmosphere to allow the pineal gland to be able to function.

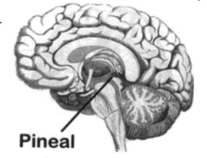

Pineal

This blend can also help decalcify the pineal gland and trigger vivid dreams, which is a sign of restful sleep.

Vibrant Blue Oils **SLEEP**™ blend and **CALM**™ blend work well to calm the body and the mind before bed.

Staying Asleep

Nighttime waking, awakening shortly after falling asleep or waking up throughout the night, can often be attributed to:

1. Blood sugar issues
2. Liver and Gallbladder overload
3. Hormonal issues

Blood Sugar Sleep Issues

Waking up in the middle of the night and feeling so wide awake that you could go clean the kitchen can suggest blood sugar issues.

If blood glucose levels drop too low during the night, the body releases the adrenal hormone epinephrine which spurs the liver to convert its stores of glycogen into glucose, raising blood glucose levels. This pattern of the body overreacting to nighttime low blood sugar is also known as the "rebound" effect or the Somogyi effect, named after researcher who first described it.

The connection between sleep and blood sugar issues goes beyond the obvious fact that when you are tired, you will crave sugar and carbohydrates for quick energy. Researchers at Boston University School of Medicine found that as the amount of sleep decreases, blood sugar increases, escalating the issue. The study found that people who slept less than six hours a night experienced blood sugar problems, compared to those who slept for eight hours or more.

This has to do in part with burning sugar versus fat for fuel. Humans are designed to burn fat during the sleep cycle because it burns long and slow, like a log on a campfire, in contrast to sugar and carbs which burn quickly, more like kindling on fire. Because of undetected blood sugar issues, many people never go into fat metabolism during the night. Instead, the body attempts to burn sugar and carbs until the supply runs out, causing blood sugar to plummet. This then triggers a epinephrine response, which, of course, can wake you up and make it tough to fall back to sleep. Many find themselves stuck in this vicious cycle of sleep deprivation raising blood sugar, and unstable blood sugar, in turn, compromising quality sleep.

Symptoms of Blood Sugar Night Waking

If you have two or more of the symptoms below, you might consider essential oils to support your blood sugar.

- ❑ Awaken hours after going to bed
- ❑ Find it difficult to go back to sleep
- ❑ Crave coffee or sweets in the afternoon
- ❑ Feel sleepy or have energy dips in afternoon
- ❑ Feel fatigued after meals
- ❑ Need stimulants such as coffee after meals
- ❑ Feel like skipping breakfast
- ❑ Slow starter in the morning
- ❑ Chronic low back pain, worse with fatigue
- ❑ Chronic fatigue, or get drowsy often

Essential Oils for Staying Asleep (Blood Sugar)

If you wake up in the middle of the night due to blood sugar issues, the following essential oils may be helpful:

PANCREAS™: The pancreas is responsible for moving glucose out of the bloodstream and into the cells. If blood sugar falls too low while you are sleeping, the body releases an emergency surge of epinephrine which spurs the liver to convert its stores of glycogen into glucose, raising blood glucose levels. The epinephrine surge feels like a kick of adrenaline and is what wakes you up. It is the job of the pancreas to kick into high gear to return blood sugar levels to normal. Supporting the pancreas in this effort with Vibrant Blue Oils **PANCREAS™** blend helps return the body to balance more quickly so you can fall back asleep more easily. I often leave the **PANCREAS™** blend on my nightstand table. Just smelling the **PANCREAS™** blend can help balance the pancreas enough to allow me to fall back asleep naturally.

Night Waking—Liver/Gallbladder Overload

According to Chinese Medicine, each organ has a time of the day/night where it does its thing, and waking between 1 a.m. and 3 a.m. is "liver time." During the night, the liver is busy rebuilding the body and cleansing it of accumulated toxins. The liver is most active between 1 a.m. and 3 a.m., often peaking at 3 a.m. When you wake at this time, it often reflects an overload in the body's ability to detoxify from toxins or emotions like anger, frustration, or resentment. Unlike blood sugar night waking, liver and gallbladder-trigger awakenings are often accompanied by a feeling of grogginess, and many find it easier to fall back asleep.

Symptoms of Liver-Related Night Waking

The liver filters and detoxifies any harmful substances from the blood while we sleep. If too many toxins accumulate and the liver is fatigued or overburdened, it might present with symptoms like:

- ❑ Waking up between 1 and 3 a.m.
- ❑ Becoming sick or easily intoxicated when drinking wine
- ❑ Easily hung over when drinking wine
- ❑ Long-term use of prescription/recreational drugs
- ❑ Sensitivity to smells, like tobacco smoke
- ❑ Pain under the right side of rib cage
- ❑ Hemorrhoids or varicose veins
- ❑ Chronic fatigue or fibromyalgia

If you recognize yourself in several of these symptoms, Vibrant Blue Oils **LIVER**™ blend might be helpful to apply before bed and during the night when you wake up.

Liver Emotions

The liver also stores and releases emotional toxins, like feelings of anger, frustration, or resentment, which might present with symptoms like:

- ❑ Feeling irritable or impatient
- ❑ Inappropriate anger, including angry outbursts
- ❑ Over-reactivity, "flying off the handle," or having a difficult time letting things go
- ❑ Feelings of not feeling heard, not feeling loved, not being recognized, inability to be honest with yourself and others
- ❑ Experience of resentment, frustration, or bitterness
- ❑ Can be judgmental, overly critical, fault-finding, or complaining
- ❑ Feeling the need to control situations; domineering or bossy

If you recognize yourself in several of these symptoms, Vibrant Blue Oils **LIVER SUPPORT**™ blend might be helpful to apply before bed and during the night when you wake up. **LIVER SUPPORT**™ helps the body detoxify from emotions like anger, frustration, or resentment that might pop up in the middle of the night and prevent restful sleep.

Gallbladder

The gallbladder concentrates the bile to help break down fat and carry toxins out of the body. If the bile becomes too thick, it doesn't flow as well, and toxins don't move out of the system as efficiently, resulting in reabsorption of toxins like old hormones. If the gallbladder is fatigued or overburdened, it might present with symptoms like:

- ❑ Waking up between 1 and 3 a.m.
- ❑ Pain between the shoulder blades
- ❑ Stomach feels upset by greasy foods
- ❑ Avoiding eating fatty food
- ❑ Stools are greasy, shiny, or float in the toilet
- ❑ Nausea or motion sickness
- ❑ Dry skin, itchy feet, or peeling skin on the feet
- ❑ Mild headache over eyes

If you recognize yourself in several of these symptoms, Vibrant Blue Oils **GALLBLADDER**™ blend might be helpful to apply before bed and during the night when you wake up.

Night Waking Due to Hormonal Issues

Hormonal ups and downs of menstruation, pregnancy, and midlife fluctuations can impact sleep. For example, the hormone progesterone promotes restful sleep, and a drop in estrogen can leave you more vulnerable to stress. Similar to blood sugar events, a rush of cortisol can cause hot flashes that alert your mind and wake you up.

Symptoms of Night Waking Hormonal Issues

- ❏ Cracked and dry heels
- ❏ Libido missing
- ❏ Rapid weight gain that won't budge
- ❏ Irregular periods, intense PMS, hot flashes or other menopausal symptoms
- ❏ Feeling moody, irritable, weepy or have unstable or unpredictable moods
- ❏ Hair loss at the crown of your head, or growth on the chin or other weird places
- ❏ Hair feels dry and "crispy"
- ❏ Skin looks crepe-y and hangs off cheeks or chin.
- ❏ Fat accumulating in new places—under arms, muffin-top, pectorals, or knees
- ❏ High cholesterol

If you recognize yourself in 2 or more of the symptoms above, you might consider essential oils to support your hormones, like Vibrant Blue Oils **HORMONE BALANCE**™ blend.

Essential Oils for Hormonal Balances

For nighttime waking due to hormonal issues, consider supporting the endocrine system and hypothalamus, which sends and receives the clear messages from the body necessary to facilitate appropriate hormonal responses. Also, excess estrogen can make the bile from the gallbladder too thick and less able to efficiently detoxify excess hormones. **GALLBLADDER**™ and **ESTROGEN BALANCE**™ oils can help return the body to balance.

HYPOTHALAMUS™– The hypothalamus is a pearl size region of the brain located just above the brainstem that serves as the control center for the entire endocrine system, including all your hormones and your adrenals. The hypothalamus determines how much cortisol is in the blood, so balancing the hypothalamus can help manage cortisol spikes. The **HYPOTHALAMUS**™ blend supports the brain to send and receive the messages from the body necessary to facilitate appropriate hormonal responses.

Excess estrogen can make the bile from the gallbladder too thick and less able to efficiently detoxify excess hormones. **GALLBLADDER**™ helps mobilize the toxins out of the body. Similarly, **ESTROGEN BALANCE**™ supports the optimal balance of estrogen with progesterone for optimal liver function and the gentle mobilization and detoxification of excess estrogen. Apply either or both over the gallbladder (on the right side of the body under the breast) to help support hormonal imbalances and more restful sleep.

Other Suggestions to Improve Sleep

Reduce Exposure to Artificial Light—Artificial light from computers, phones, and other electronic devices disrupts the body's natural ability to determine light from dark, which disturbs the circadian rhythm and throws off your sleep. The blue light emitted from alarm clocks and other digital devices also suppresses melatonin production.

Turn off Wi-Fi in the house.

Make the bedroom as dark as possible. Use blackout shades to make your bedroom pitch black and cover or turn off all devices that glow or give off any light (including digital alarm clocks).

Don't be too full—or too hungry. Some people sleep better after eating a light dinner. This is especially true for those with digestive issues. Others—like those with a tendency toward hypoglycemia—do better with a snack before bed (and possibly even during the night).

Go to bed earlier. You've heard the saying "an hour before midnight is worth two hours after." It turns out there is some truth to that.

Chapter 5

Stress

S tress is the body's reaction to potentially dangerous situations, real or perceived. Any physical, emotional, psychological, or environmental stimulus that the mind perceives as a threat triggers a stress response to supply the body with the energy it needs to respond.

A *stressor* can be any physical, emotional, psychological or environmental threat that can knock us out of homeostatic balance.

Examples of Stressors

Physical Stress: Anything stressing the physical body—including physical injuries such as a headache, chronic inflammation, pain, scars or surgeries, structural misalignment like a clenched jaw, or even physical exercise—can stress our systems.

Environmental Stress: Toxins in the environment—including mold, pesticides, pollution, chemicals in the home (cleaning products, skin care), chlorine or fluoride in tap water, food additives or preservatives, vaccines, electromagnetic emissions from cell phones, Wi-Fi, computers, cell towers, or smart meters—can add to our stress load.

Psychological or External Emotional Stress: Stressful experiences like the death of loved one, divorce, surgery, financial hardship, bad relationships, or work environment, and other conditions that entail feelings of helplessness

Internal Emotional Stress: The body cannot differentiate a perceived threat based on repetitive thoughts and emotions from an actual physical stress. As a result, prolonged repetitive negative thought patterns—such as those surrounding abandonment, anger, anxiety, betrayal, controlling, depression, fear, grief, guilt, hopelessness, jealousy, lack of control, nervousness, overwhelm, panic, poor boundaries, resentment, sadness, self-abuse, shame or humiliation, shock, sorrow, trauma, feeling unsupported or taken for granted, worry, and unworthiness—can keep us locked in a constant stress response.

Physiological Stress: The process of running the body itself can contribute to stress levels. For example, any low-level infection, fever, sensitivities to foods like gluten or dairy, blood sugar imbalances, vitamin or mineral deficiencies, imbalances in your gut flora, dysbiosis, a leaky gut or maldigestion, parasites, constipation, sleep deficiency, dehydration, digestive, cardiovascular or skin issues, autoimmunity, liver toxicity, or kidney stress adds to the cumulative stress level.

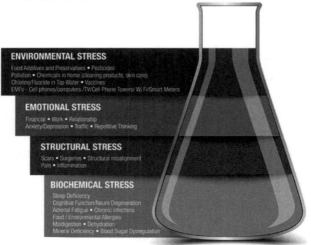

Interplay Between Stressors

Stresses are additive and cumulative. The volume of stresses, the intensity of each stress, and the frequency and duration of time combine to form a total stress load. In other words, the more you layer on, the more likely you are to overwhelm your system.

Imagine a cup of water that is completely full. Even a drop of additional water will cause the cup to overflow. But when the cup is less full, it would take more water to cause a spill. Stress in the body is like that. Removing small stressors can have a big impact. Even tidying your environment and purging items that you no longer need or use can be a powerful stress relief. It removes stressful clutter, and every little stress that you can remove adds up.

That said, there is an interplay between physiological imbalances, such as the stress load, blood sugar regulation, detoxification, and gut inflammation. When imbalanced, they all contribute to the total stress load of the body. For example, dysregulation in any of these systems can trigger a stress response:

➤ **Blood sugar imbalances** can trigger a cortisol response and increases stress.
➤ **Negative emotions** or thoughts can trigger a stress reaction in the body.
➤ **Leaky Gut:** Toxins or pathogens entering the blood via the gut put stress on the body.
➤ **Digestion:** Malabsorption of nutrients also depletes the body of the vitamins and minerals necessary to chemically support the stress response.
➤ **Detoxification:** When toxins aren't removed from the body, they recirculate and become a stressor.

The physiological stress from the process of running the body often accounts for at least 30 percent of the body's total stress load. It is, therefore, important when attempting to reduce your stress load to also look at balancing these physiological functions. To assess your stress load, go to www.vibrantblueoils.com/bookbonus.

What Does Stress Do to the Body?

Stress triggers a domino effect in the body to go on high alert "fight-or-flight" and free up all available energy and resources to escape the perceived threat. This is known as a stress response, and it activates both the nervous system and the endocrine system

The body's first line of defense against stress is the sympathetic branch of the autonomic nervous system. In the sympathetic "fight-or-flight" state, the body kicks into survival mode, releasing hormones like adrenaline and rushing blood to your brain, heart, and muscles to help you flee from immediate danger. Once the danger has passed, the body is designed to drop back into the parasympathetic state, which brings the body back to normal, relaxed functioning.

In other words, the sympathetic response is ideal for short and acute responses to stress.

More constant stress can keep you locked in the "fight-or-flight" sympathetic state and locked out of the "rest-and-digest" parasympathetic state. For more information on the parasympathetic state, go to Chapter 3.

HPA Axis Stress Response

Stress also triggers a complex hormonal cascade in the endocrine system, involving the hypothalamus, the pituitary, and the adrenals and known as the hypothalamic-pituitary-adrenal axis.

In addition to controlling our reaction to stress, the HPA axis and interactions between these organs regulate many of our body's processes, including digestion, the immune system, cardiovascular and respiratory systems, detoxification, circadian rhythms, thyroid function, mood and emotions, sexuality, and energy storage and expenditure.

The general hormonal cascade flows like this:

> The hypothalamus releases corticotrophin-releasing hormone (**CRH)**
> This signals the **anterior pituitary** to secrete **ACTH** (adrenocorticotropic hormone).
> **ACTH** stimulates the **adrenal cortex** to produce **cortisol** to raise the sugar in your bloodstream to increase energy for stress response.

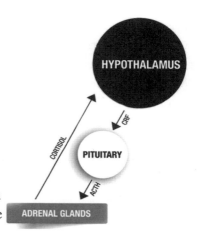

These interactions continue until your hormones reach the levels that your body needs, and then a series of chemical reactions known as the negative feedback loop begins to switch them off. For example, the **hypothalamus** receives signals when cortisol levels are sufficient and inhibits **CRH** release.

Now that you understand the general overview, I will dive more deeply into each organ function:

The hypothalamus is a pearl-size region of the brain located just above the brainstem that serves as the control center for neural and hormonal messages received from/sent to the body, including all hormonal messages for the endocrine, stress, and digestive systems. It brings together the **nervous system** (electrical signals to communicate to the nervous system) and **endocrine systems** (hormonal signals) to oversee the body's homeostasis.

It achieves this by sending hormonal signals to the organs, then adjusting its response based on the incoming signals from the organs. For example, it will trigger the pituitary gland to release hormones directing the adrenal glands to release the stress hormone cortisol.

When sufficient levels of cortisol are in the system, it is supposed to inhibit the hypothalamus and pituitary (so they stop sending signals to produce more cortisol)! This is known as a negative feedback loop, which only works when accurate feedback is received.

The hypothalamus has to function optimally, both in its ability to send and receive messages, for the cascade of hormones to fall into balance. To this point, the ability of the hypothalamus to receive clear messages from the body is critical, as all outgoing endocrine and neural signals are based on the clarity of these incoming signals. Chronic and prolonged stress can take a toll on the hypothalamus and its ability to send and receive optimal signals.

When the hypothalamus is out of balance, it can negatively impact:

- ➢ Adrenal function
- ➢ Thyroid function
- ➢ Hunger impulses
- ➢ The ability to handle stress
- ➢ All endocrine function (including the sexual organs)

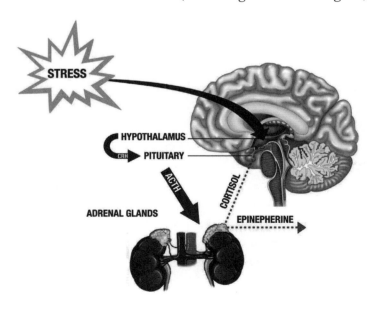

Symptoms of Hypothalamus Imbalance

❑ Body temperature problems and cold intolerance
❑ Constipation
❑ Depressed mood
❑ Excessive thirst/frequent urination
❑ Fatigue
❑ Hair or skin changes
❑ Mental slowing
❑ Menstrual cycle changes
❑ Weight gain
❑ Lowered libido

The Pituitary

The pituitary is an endocrine gland about the size of a pea located at the base of the brain, just below the hypothalamus, that regulates several physiological processes—stress, growth, reproduction, lactation, and water metabolism. It plays a key hormonal role in the body, releasing appropriate hormones, which affect downstream glands. It also receives feedback from downstream glands known as the negative feedback system and responds accordingly.

The Adrenal Glands

The small, triangular-shaped adrenal glands situated on top of the kidneys regulate the body's stress response by secreting key hormones, like cortisol and adrenaline (epinephrine), that regulate energy production and storage, increase blood sugar, depress immune function, reduce inflammation, increase heart rate, increase muscle tone, and other processes that enable you to rapidly respond to stress. They mobilize the body's responses to every kind of stress. Every stress response is an adrenal response, including signaling the kidney to retain sodium, which is needed for stress responses.

The adrenal glands release many hormones, but cortisol is the key hormone in supporting stress responses, as it increases blood sugar to support the body's increased energy needs during a stress response and also depresses immune, detoxification, regeneration, and digestion to conserve energy for the stress response.

The health and resilience of the adrenals (along with the hypothalamus and hippocampus) help to determine our tolerance to stress.

When the adrenals are dealing with a lot of stress, they either:

➢ Slip into overdrive and attempt to over-function, a condition known as hyper-cortisol, or
➢ Become so depleted that they are unable to release or produce the hormones that you need to react to a stressful situation, commonly referred to as adrenal fatigue.

Symptoms of Hyper-Cortisol Adrenals:

❑ Tendency to be a "night person"
❑ Difficulty falling asleep
❑ Tendency to be keyed up, have trouble calming down
❑ Blood pressure above 120/80
❑ Feeling wired or jittery after drinking coffee
❑ Clenching or grinding teeth
❑ Calm on the outside, troubled on the inside
❑ Arthritic tendencies
❑ Perspire easily
❑ Tendency to sprain ankles or "shin splints"

Symptoms of Adrenal Fatigue:

- ❑ Slow starter in the morning
- ❑ Fatigue that is not relieved by sleep
- ❑ Chronic low back pain, worse with fatigue
- ❑ Becoming dizzy when standing up suddenly
- ❑ Pain after or difficulty maintaining manipulative correction
- ❑ Craving salty foods or salt foods before tasting
- ❑ Afternoon yawning or headache
- ❑ Tendency to need sunglasses

Different supplements are often recommended for hyper versus fatigued adrenals, but the main goal is to return the adrenals to balance. Essential oils can play a key role here.

Essential Oils to Support Stress

PARASYMPATHETIC™: If you are stuck in the sympathetic-dominant state, you are never able to rest, digest, and heal. To help stimulate the parasympathetic response, apply Vibrant Blue Oils **PARASYMPATHETIC™** blend to the vagal nerve (behind the earlobe and up one inch on the mastoid bone). For more aggressive vagal stimulation, you can also apply at the base of the skull (where you feel a small indent). Apply before meals to optimize digestion and up to six times daily to help reset the body into the parasympathetic state.

HYPOTHALAMUS™: Helps balance the hypothalamus, the control center for all hormones, controlling the endocrine system, digestive system, and nervous systems. When the hypothalamus functions optimally, the cascade of hormones falls into balance. Apply one drop to the forehead above the third eye (above the nose between eyebrows and hairline).

ADRENAL™: The adrenal glands help determine and regulate the body's stress response by secreting hormones like adrenaline and cortisol. Prolonged periods of stress can deplete our reserves of these hormones and exhaust the adrenal glands. Applying Vibrant Blue Oils **ADRENAL™** blend over the adrenal glands (back of the body, one fist up from the 12th rib), may help to increase the body's ability to adapt to stress and maintain healthy adrenal function.

KIDNEY SUPPORT™ for fear: The sympathetic nervous system is the "fight-or-flight" system. It is the body's response to fear. Anything that creates fear, whether it is listening to the news, watching a scary movie, or any other frightening situation, can contribute to sympathetic-dominance symptoms. In Chinese medicine, feelings of fear and paranoia can be held in the kidneys, impairing their function. Applying Vibrant Blue Oils **KIDNEY SUPPORT™** over the kidneys (on the back of the body the size of a fist starting at the bottom rib), over the forehead, the back of neck, or around the outside of the earlobes can help you flow through fear.

LIVER SUPPORT™ for anger: Many people with sympathetic dominance are quite angry underneath. They may be spiritually advanced individuals who are having trouble handling the world. It can also be for all sorts of other reasons, such as childhood traumas. For many in a sympathetic-dominance pattern, anger often presents an adrenal response to fear projected onto others. Vibrant Blue Oils **LIVER SUPPORT™** helps support the release of emotions, including persistent irritation, impatience, resentment or frustration, being critical of yourself or others, control issues, an inability to express your feelings, feelings of not feeling heard, not feeling loved, not being recognized or appreciated. For more tips on how to detoxify emotions, refer to Chapter 6.

CALM™ for anxiety: This gentle blend is ideal for alleviating anxiety, a racing heartbeat, feelings of overwhelm, and promoting calm and relaxation. This is a very gentle blend that may be applied over the heart or massaged along the outside of ears. It is a wonderful blend for children and may be massaged on the bottoms of the feet before bed, especially after an overactive or stressful day.

For more information on balancing environmental toxins, refer to Chapter 9 on Detoxification.

Chronic and prolonged stress triggers the adrenal glands to release excess cortisol at night, throwing off our body's natural cortisol/melatonin rhythm. For information on balancing Sleep, refer to Chapter 4.

Chapter 6

Emotions

Our emotions and thought patterns can play a major role in our ability to heal. For example, negative emotions, like fear, anger, and grief, can keep us locked in a state of constant and chronic stress; while positive emotions like love and gratitude can help amplify our healing. Essential oils can positively and immediately impact the emotional centers of the brain, making them potent tools to help your body feel better and to help your mind feel happier!

Emotions and the Body's Stress Response

Patterns of constant stress often stem not solely from stressors in the present moment, like a job, relationship, or finances, but from deep-seated emotions and their resulting thought patterns. This realization led to a profound shift in my healing. I've also seen such an awareness facilitate healing in many of my clients. You see, memories of past trauma or fears and worries about the future often trigger stress. The body cannot differentiate between physical stress and emotional or thought-driven stress. It responds to both with the same cascade of stress hormones.

In other words, stressful thoughts or emotions trigger a stress response in the body. And a body in stress cannot heal. Lissa Rankin writes about this in her book, *The Fear Cure*, noting that fear drives most stress. This fear can come from both physical threats and emotional thought patterns.

"Fear from physical threats is a survival mechanism meant to protect us," Rankin writes. "It throws us into the flight-or-fight sympathetic response necessary to survive. A physical fear response is triggered if our car spins out of control on a highway or we get robbed at gunpoint. This kind of fear is critical to our safety and survival. Emotional or thought-driven fears are based on anxiety, worry, and resulting thought patterns about all the things that could go wrong in an imaginary future."

Unfortunately, the body and its stress response cannot tell the difference between a physical threat and emotional fear. We release the same flood of stress hormones, like cortisol and adrenaline, in both cases. For those of us who suffer from anxiety, worry, or fear, this often means that our bodies can get stuck in the vicious cycle of a constant stress response. Every time the brain, specifically the amygdala, responds to a fear-based stress, it becomes more sensitized and reactive to other apparent threats.

As the amygdala also helps to form memories, a chronic stress response can amplify feelings of anxiety and fear. On a chemical level, this constant exposure to stress hormones like cortisol can weaken neuronal synapses in the brain and inhibit the formation of new ones, impacting our ability to make new memories.

"This can result in a chronically fearful and anxious feeling with no real memory of why we are even afraid," notes Rankin. She explains that our sensitized amygdala programs these fearful experiences into implicit memory, while our weakened hippocampus fails to record new explicit memories. Even long after the threat is over, anything that triggers this fearful response, consciously or unconsciously, stimulates the thalamus, which stimulates the amygdala and retrieves the fearful memory from the hippocampus and suddenly the body goes into hyper-drive. Once triggered, the physical reaction that follows is a warning system malfunction, alerting us to dangers that don't actually threaten us. This false fear is nothing more than a thought, but it leads to a potent stress response that affects not just your mind but your body. As a result of this warning system malfunction, fear can take over the nervous system, contributing to phobias, post-traumatic stress reactions, anxiety disorders, depression, and other psychiatric conditions. No matter how motivated you are to heal, you just can't will yourself to be free of these kinds of fears, because the fear stems from unconscious processes and hooks into the most primal part of the nervous system.

Fortunately, essential oils can directly alter the emotional centers of the brain. When inhaled, the volatile compounds of essential oils travel into the nasal passages, where they directly trigger the brain's limbic system (the emotion and memory center). This immediate reaction bypasses the brain's intellectual, logical centers.

This direct access makes sense, as the sense of smell evolved to support our survival. It helps us determine what food is healthy to eat or rotten; it helps us detect predators or dangers like fire. In fact, studies have shown that odor learning begins before birth when flavor compounds from the maternal diet get incorporated into amniotic fluid and are ingested by the developing fetus. Studies monitoring mothers' consumption of distinctive smelling substances such as garlic, alcohol, or cigarette smoke during pregnancy found that their infants preferred these smells compared to infants who had not been exposed to these scents.

Limbic System

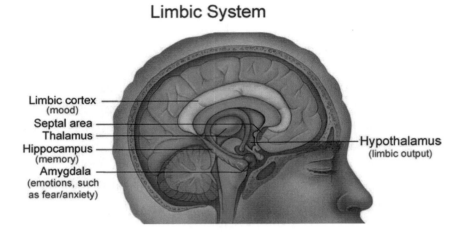

Limbic cortex (mood)
Septal area
Thalamus
Hippocampus (memory)
Amygdala (emotions, such as fear/anxiety)
Hypothalamus (limbic output)

Emotions as a Warning Signal

Some believe that emotions can cause physical discomfort, like a nervous stomach, and the key to relieving the physical symptoms is to work on resolving the underlying emotional cause. In my life and my practice, I have found that when a physical complaint or discomfort does not improve with conventional dietary and lifestyle support, it is often related to an emotion wanting to be recognized and released. Interestingly, once the underlying emotional issue is identified, released, and healed, the physical discomfort seems to subside.

You might consider the lesson that specific emotions carry. Once you learn that lesson, the emotion that accompanies it and any corresponding physical discomfort will often pass. For example, the attempt to control a situation is often related to fear that the situation may not work out the way you have in mind.

I struggled with this fear. I would try to plan every moment of a vacation, down to the last detail, making our vacations feel stressful and rushed. In my effort to work through this issue, I decided when planning a recent vacation to let go of control and be open to the natural flow. The most amazing thing happened!

Not only did we hit all the highlights I had hoped to see, but we also made room for some unexpected and insanely fun experiences that my new flexibility allowed us to enjoy.

I invite you to consider viewing emotions as an opportunity to let go of hurt or negative thought patterns and emotions so you can learn from them or let them pass. I completely understand that an emotion can be so painful or intense that you do not know how to work through it. But it may be stored in the body, often in the corresponding organ or system, and then you replay it over and over in your mind, often to the detriment of vibrant health.

How Emotions Impact the Physical Body

Chinese medicine proposes that negative emotions cause a disruption in the body's energy system, often in connection to certain meridians and organs in the body. This can create stuck energy and impede an organ's ability to heal.

The word "emotions" can translate as "energy-in-motion." Emotion is the experience of energy moving through the body, signifying that emotions are meant for us to experience and move through. This emotional energy works at a higher speed than thought. Thought and images can take seconds or even minutes to evoke a memory, while smell can evoke a memory in milliseconds. Forgotten memories and suppressed emotions can wreak havoc in our lives; often being the unsourced causes of depression, anxiety, and fears. Essential oils can help release emotions stored in the body or energy field.

When we lack the tools or the support to move through these emotions or thought patterns, they can get trapped in the body as concentrated and condensed fields of energy, often in the corresponding organ area, disrupting the body's innate intelligence and energy flow.

Releasing those emotions and thought patterns can often help heal the associated organ.

Essential Oils for Emotional Support

Essential oils, with their ability to directly access areas of the brain associated with emotions and memory, are uniquely suited to help us modify thought patterns and their related emotions so we can move forward in our progress toward healing.

In 1989, Dr.Joseph Ledoux from New York University discovered that the amygdala plays a much more critical role in the storage and release of emotional traumas than previously believed. Dr. LeDoux's research was the first to recognize that the amygdala triggers an emotional reaction before the thinking brain has fully processed nerve signals. In other words, emotional reactions and emotional memories can be formed AND RELEASED without any conscious, cognitive participation at all.

This compelling breakthrough in understanding how the brain processes emotion, coupled with olfactory research by Professor Rachel S. Herz of Brown University, holds tremendous promise for the use of essential oils in helping to release negative emotion patterns unconsciously. "The olfactory bulbs are part of the limbic system and directly connect with limbic structures that process emotion (the amygdala) and associative learning (the hippocampus). No other sensory system has this type of intimate link with the neural areas of emotion and associative learning, therefore there is a strong neurological basis for why odors trigger emotional connections," wrote Herz in a *Scientific American* article, "Do scents affect people's moods or work performance?" In a follow-up research paper, Herz wrote: "The emotional power of smell-triggered memory has an intensity unequaled by sight and sound-triggered ones." Since sound is not as effective as smell for releasing memory trauma, talking about your problems in therapy or group settings might not heal the underlying emotions as effectively as releasing them through the use of aromatic essential oils.

Use the Breath to Release Past Hurts

When you detoxify the liver, it is not enough simply to mobilize the toxins. You need to ensure that they leave the body and that you replenish the depleted organs with nourishing food and energy. This is true of emotional toxins, too. You want them to leave the body's energy field and replenish it with appropriate emotions. The combination of breath, essential oils, and affirmations (if you are comfortable adding them) helps release and repair emotional blocks, diminishing the pattern of the negative emotions and thoughts and replacing them with more positive options. This helps to balance the nervous system and enhance and open the energetic field for optimal healing and vibrant health. Adding other modalities, like tapping (Emotional Freedom Techniques), can be helpful too.

Release Emotions with Breath

1. RECALL: Focus on the negative emotions or repetitive thought patterns that you would like to release. Try to recall where you first experienced this emotion or thought pattern

2. VALIDATE: Validate yourself, the experience, and the emotions you are feeling.

3. RELEASE: Deeply inhale the smell of the oil while you concentrate on the past hurt or emotion. Exhale for between three and seven breaths, allowing the negative emotions to flow out of you.

4. REPLACE: Fill the negative space of the released the emotion with a positive intention or affirmation

First, focus on the negative emotions or repetitive thought patterns that you would like to release. You can do this by speaking your concern out loud to yourself in front of a mirror, the moon, or a trusted friend. If you can, try to dig deep into your emotional memory and recall where you might have first experienced this emotion or thought pattern—perhaps somewhere in early childhood. Validate yourself, this experience, and the emotions you are feeling. You have every right to feel anger, fear, grief, shame, guilt... you name it. You are entitled to those feelings, but those feelings are no longer serving you. So it is time to release them.

In this process, the exhale releases the hurts of the past. Therefore, the deeper you breathe while smelling oils and the more forceful the out breath, the sooner the emotion is released. My favorite technique is this: taking a deep breath, slowly inhale the oil, and then exhale for between three and seven breaths. You will know that the oil is working when you stop smelling it. It is also important to fill that gap with a positive emotion, like love.

Deeply inhale the smell of the oil while you concentrate on the past hurt or emotion. Acknowledge those intense emotions, and then as you exhale, allow them to flow out of you. If tears flow as well, just allow it, as tears help release old hormones from the body.

Once you feel that you have released the emotion to the best of your ability, you can then fill the negative space with a positive affirmation. I have suggested affirmations for each blend, based on Louise Hay's suggestions in *You Can Heal Your Life*, but you are encouraged to replace them with anything that calls to your heart.

The process of instilling a positive affirmation is the same: inhale the oil for three to seven breaths and concentrate on the positive affirmation as if you are breathing it into your system. Hold the breath and let the positive affirmation settle into your body. You might physically feel your system relax and return to balance. When you are ready, exhale slowly.

You can repeat this breathing exercise as often you need it, knowing that the intensity of the emotional memory will fade the more you release it with the oils and your breath. Do note that since we are all bio-individual, experiences may vary from person to person.

Essential Oils for Emotional Clearing

To stimulate the amygdala with the sense of smell and help support the gentle release of emotional trauma and old thought patterns, consider the following emotion balance blends designed to support the release of emotions and the associated organs:

- ➤ Fear with **KIDNEY SUPPORT**™
- ➤ Anger with **LIVER SUPPORT**™
- ➤ Anxiety with **ADRENAL**™ or **CALM**™
- ➤ Grief with **LUNG SUPPORT**™
- ➤ Trauma with **BLADDER SUPPORT**™
- ➤ Depression or loneliness with **UPLIFT**™
- ➤ Worry with **SPLEEN SUPPORT**™
- ➤ Control issues with **LARGE INTESTINE SUPPORT**™
- ➤ Boundary issues with **SMALL INTESTINE SUPPORT**™
- ➤ Speaking your truth with **THYROID SUPPORT**™

BLADDER SUPPORT™ for Trauma

In Chinese medicine, the bladder is considered a storehouse for emotions, managing emotional reserves and overflow. When you feel internally empty of reserves, everything seems to be too much to handle, uncertain, and frightening. Similarly, when emotions are overflowing, you can feel awash in an internal torrent, drowning, out of control, and driven to desperation.

Often these overwhelming emotions feel like too much to handle in the moment, so you store them in the bladder until you can process and move through them. Applying 2 to 3 drops of **BLADDER SUPPORT**™ over the bladder (just above and behind the pubic bone), directly over areas of trauma or abuse, over the forehead, or around the outside of earlobes allows you

103

to let go of the negative past and release the emotional trauma from the body. It assists in overcoming feelings of despair and a sense of being pushed over the edge.

As you release any negative emotional debris stored in the bladder with **BLADDER SUPPORT™**, you might consider supporting the body as it returns to balance with the following affirmation to overcome trauma:

I comfortably and easily release the old and welcome the new into my life. I am safe.

CALM™ or ADRENAL™ for Anxiety

Any stress in the body can trigger the adrenal glands to release the stress hormones adrenaline or cortisol. A prolonged stress response can throw the body out of balance. The **ADRENAL™** blend is designed to balance the extremes, calming the adrenals when too much cortisol is released and supporting them during periods of adrenal fatigue. This blend can be very powerful when smelled, helping to reduce anxiety. You can also apply it over the adrenal glands (on the lower mid-back, one fist above the 12th rib on each side). This blend can be hot, so definitely dilute before using topically in the beginning. Similarly, **CALM™** helps alleviate anxiety, worries, a racing heartbeat, and feelings of overwhelm when applied over the heart, the nape of the neck, wrists, on the forehead or the outside of ears. The gentle blend is extremely effective in calming active or hard-to-manage children, especially when applied over the heart or on the bottoms of the feet before bed.

Other blends can help support anxiety, including **PARASYMPATHETIC™** will trigger the body's relaxation response as a counterbalance to the "fight-or-flight" stress response (See Chapter 5 for more). **HYPOTHALAMUS™** can also help balance stress hormones to reduce anxiety.

As you release your anxiety with CALM™ or ADRENAL™, you might consider supporting the body as it returns to balance with the following affirmation to overcome trauma:

With every breath, I release the anxiety within me, and I become more and more calm.

KIDNEY SUPPORT™ for Fear

Any shift in the body can trigger a fear response. Feelings of fear and paranoia can be held in the kidneys, impairing their function. In Chinese medicine, the kidneys are associated with emotions of fear. They are also considered the seat of courage and willpower.

In the physical body, the kidneys filter blood, regulate the balance of fluids, and remove water-soluble waste products. They control the volume, composition, and pressure of fluids in all the cells. Blood flows through the kidneys at its highest pressure, filtering out toxins and directing nourishing materials to where they are needed. Water is symbolic of the unconscious, our emotion, and of that which we do not understand and that which we fear.

Balancing the kidneys by topically applying KIDNEY SUPPORT™ over the kidneys (starting at the 12th rib in the area about the size of a fist) or on the forehead may help dispel fear and assist in feeling safe.

As you release your fear with KIDNEY SUPPORT™, you might consider supporting the body as it returns to balance with the following affirmation:

I dissolve my fear with ease. I am safe.

LARGE INTESTINE ™ to Release Control

The large intestine lets go of those things that don't serve us.

Physically, it lets go of waste after the upper digestive system has taken all the necessary nutrients out of the food we eat. Emotionally, it allows the body to let go of patterns of negative thinking, destructive emotions, and spiritual blockages that prevent you from being your best.

Compromised large intestine energy presents as having a hard time moving on from difficult situations, or holding onto emotions that harm or fail to serve. This holding on can manifest as an unwillingness to share emotions or be open with others; the phenomenon of "bottling up" emotions for years very often leads to chronic constipation.

Apply 2 to 3 drops of **LARGE INTESTINE SUPPORT**™ over the large intestine, around the ears, on the forehead or on the bottoms of the feet to assist with releasing control through transitions when emotionally stuck or changing course in life. The blend may help ease the feelings of loss, add balance, and create a sense of security so you can release the need to control

As you release your need to control with **LARGE INTESTINE SUPPORT**™, you might consider supporting the body as it returns to balance with the following affirmation:

I easily release that which I no longer need. The past is over. I am free.

LIVER SUPPORT™ for Anger

The liver plays over 500 roles in the body, including digesting vital nutrients and storing them as energy. It safely mobilizes, filters, and eliminates emotional and physical toxins from the body. Energetically, the liver is associated with the smooth flow of energy, blood, and mental and emotional stress through the body.

In Chinese medicine, the liver is often associated with anger. If the liver is not able to detoxify stress-related hormones, their re-circulation can result in radical mood shifts and inappropriate angry behavior. Similarly, thought-produced toxins may lead to extreme feelings of anger and frustration.

Applying 2 to 3 drops of **LIVER SUPPORT**™ over the liver (right side of the body under the breast) or on the forehead can support the gentle release of anger, along with any other negative emotions from the cells of the liver. You can also top the blend with a castor oil pack over the liver to enhance the penetration. Inhalation is also a very helpful tool for emotional release. Just hold the bottle about an inch or two below the nose and deeply breathe in the oil to the count of six, then gently exhale just as slowly. As you exhale, imagine exhaling any anxiety, fear, or emotion you wish to move through. Repeat this for three to seven breaths. It is not uncommon to stop smelling the oil at some point during this process, as that is often indicative of the body shifting.

As you release your anger with **LIVER SUPPORT**™, you might consider supporting the body as it returns to balance with the following affirmation:

I clear and release any and all unresolved anger, rage, betrayals, or frustration from my system. I grant myself the gift of compassion and forgiveness!

LUNG SUPPORT™ for Grief

We all get a little attached to our stuff, even the negative emotions that no longer serve, and there can be a sense of grief or loss in letting go. I suspect that maybe one of the reasons so many of us cling to a bad relationship or situation that no longer serves. It is painful to move on and grow, and we have to acknowledge and work through the grief that comes with it.

The lungs are an important channel of elimination, holding grief when you are not yet ready to let go of situations or emotions that no longer serve.

They function as a fundamental source of life energy – transporting oxygen from the atmosphere into the capillaries so they can oxygenate blood—as well as an important channel of elimination—releasing carbon dioxide from the bloodstream into the atmosphere.

Feelings of grief, bereavement, regret, loss, and remorse can obstruct the ability of the lungs to accept and relinquish, impeding their function of "taking in" and "letting go." Grief that remains unresolved can become chronic and create disharmony in the lungs, weakening the lung's function of circulating oxygen around the body. When lung function is impaired, it leads to shortness of breath, fatigue, and feelings of melancholy. Sadly, many chronic respiratory diseases and conditions develop after a significant loss or bereavement.

Smelling **LUNG SUPPORT™** or gently massaging it over the lungs, around the ear lobes (which serve as reflexology points for the body and the release of many emotions) or over the forehead can help support the gentle release of grief. Allow yourself to deeply exhale any grief as you apply the blend. A normal and healthy expression of grief can be expressed as sobbing that originates deep in the lungs, including deep breaths and the expulsion of air with the sob.

As you release your grief with **LUNG SUPPORT™**, you might consider supporting the body as it returns to balance with the following affirmation:

I release my grief with ease and take in the fullness of life.

SMALL INTESTINE SUPPORT™ for Boundaries

The small intestine is the boundary center of the body. It absorbs and assimilates key nutrients while preventing harmful pathogens and toxins from entering the body.

On an emotional level, the small intestine plays a similarly discerning role, helping you to understand experiences and determine healthy and appropriate relationships and boundaries. It is also an area where you can hold deep childhood scars of rejection, abandonment or abuse; negative thoughts fueled by feelings of lack of self-worth, low self-esteem, loneliness, neglect, and anxieties about survival and success. In short, the small intestine sorts and transforms food, feelings, and ideas into useful ingredients for the body and mind. It also helps correct imbalances where you are overly in tune with others' feelings at the expense of your own.

To foster clear boundaries that are supportive and nurturing to your physical, emotional, mental, and spiritual health, apply 2 to 3 drops of **SMALL INTESTINE SUPPORT™** around the belly button in a clockwise direction. It is also helpful to apply it around the ears, starting at the bottom of the ear at the earlobes and gentle massage upward along the exterior of the ear, hitting many of the major reflexology points or on the forehead.

As you strengthen your boundaries with **SMALL INTESTINE SUPPORT™**, you might consider supporting the body as it returns to balance with the following affirmation:

I trust myself and my judgment. I easily assimilate and absorb all that I need and release the past with joy.

SPLEEN SUPPORT™ for Worry

The spleen, located in the left upper quadrant of the abdomen, acts as a filter for blood as part of the immune system. The spleen recycles old red blood cells and stores platelets and white blood cells. The spleen helps fight certain kinds of bacteria that cause pneumonia and meningitis.

According to Chinese medicine, the spleen houses the body's thoughts and intentions and is responsible for analytical thinking, memory, cognition, intelligence, and ideas. These emotions in their extreme states—over-thinking, worry, excessive mental and intellectual stimulation, or any activity that involves a lot of mental effort—can create disharmony in the spleen.If you "ruminate" and constantly obsess about life experiences, you are not "transforming" them into positive fuel to motivate taking action and move forward in life.

To assist in calming worries, easing anxiety, and balancing and stabilizing obsessive thoughts and emotions, apply 2 to 3 drops of **SPLEEN SUPPORT**™ over the spleen (left side of the body, under the breast), over the forehead or around the earlobes for emotional support.

As you release your worry with **SPLEEN SUPPORT**™, you might consider supporting the body as it returns to balance with the following affirmation:

I release worry and embrace balance. I love and approve of myself and trust the process of life to be there for me. I am safe. All is well.

THYROID SUPPORT™ for Speaking your Truth

The thyroid gland, located below the Adam's apple on the neck, coordinates the metabolism (growth and rate of function) of almost every cell in the body. It controls how quickly the body uses energy and makes proteins, and it controls the body's sensitivity to other hormones.

The thyroid relates emotionally to self-expression and the struggle to communicate. This includes speaking up for yourself as well as not suppressing your truth, failing to ask for what you want, and feeling you do not have the right to ask for what you want. Suppressed communication can give rise to feelings of humiliation, never getting to do what you want to do, or thoughts and emotions related to "your turn" in life. (i.e. "When is it going to be MY turn?")

An inability to speak your truth—including difficulty in self-expression, feeling suppressed or shut down in creative endeavors or "swallowing" or "stifling" your words to keep the peace or win people's approval—will often cause physical problems in the thyroid, mouth, and neck area around the throat.

To support clear expression and overcome feelings of humiliation, inhibition, and denial, apply 2 to 3 drops of **THYROID SUPPORT**™ over the throat or heart or around the ears.

As you speak your truth with **THYROID SUPPORT**™, you might consider supporting the body as it returns to balance with the following affirmation:

I move beyond old limitations and now allow myself to express freely and creatively.

UPLIFT™ for Depression

Depression can be paralyzing, mentally and physically. It diminishes your vitality, joy, and mental clarity. Depression can also make it challenging to heal and grow as your thoughts are integrally connected with your health and well-being.

UPLIFT™ was specially formulated with oils that assist in building courage, confidence, and self-esteem, and that return a sense of calm, joy, and peace to your life. It inspires hope in those who have temporarily lost their optimism and helps users to overcome their fear and reclaim their potential. When you have more courage to take on new things and/or change, you are better able to release old patterns that are not working for you.

It can also align the physical, mental, and emotional energies of the body when applied to shoulders, the bottoms of the feet, the outside of the ears or on the forehead.

To help alleviate depression and promote feelings of strength, courage, and protection, apply 2 to 3 drops of **UPLIFT**™ to the vagus nerve (behind the earlobe and up one inch, on the mastoid bone) and over the heart, wrists, temples, and forehead. To keep balanced and confident during the day, rub three to six drops on the bottoms of your feet each morning.

In addition to reducing negative emotions like sadness or depression, it is helpful to heighten positive emotions like those of joy and love. **HEART**™, applied over the heart, on the forehead or around the earlobes, can be very uplifting and comforting, helping to shift you back into a state of balance and joy. Similarly, **ROSE**™ is known for having a very high frequency to immediately help shift the body into a more balanced, joyful state.

As you lift the heavy energy of depression with **UPLIFT**™, you might consider supporting the body as it returns to balance with the following affirmation:

I release and clear any thoughts, emotions, and patterns that limit my ability to experience joy, love, and support. I open my heart to receiving everything that I need.

Chapter 7

Digestion

Our health depends not just on what we eat, but our ability to digest, absorb, and assimilate our nutrients. The body's digestive system performs specific tasks to keep it running smoothly.

- ➢ Stomach releases stomach acid, to digest proteins more completely.
- ➢ Pancreas releases enzymes to digest protein, carbohydrates, and fats.
- ➢ Gallbladder releases bile to break down and assimilate fat
- ➢ Small Intestine assimilates nutrients and moves food through the digestive tract.
- ➢ Large Intestine eliminates waste.

Fat, in particular, can be challenging to digest. Many popular diets contain high levels of animal protein and fat that many of us are unable to digest and assimilate properly.

A few years ago, I attended a Paleo conference where I offered free health assessments. I expected to find a very healthy population of attendees. Much to my surprise, almost every person I assessed showed signs of poor fat digestion and assimilation. While they were eating a nutrient-dense, whole food diet, much of the fat was not being properly absorbed and assimilated. When the body is not assimilating fat properly, any diet that overloads the body with dietary fat can cause more harm than good. Fortunately, topically applied essential oils can play a key supporting role in optimizing digestion.

Eating in the Parasympathetic State

Digestion is a "rest-and-digest" parasympathetic event. Our nervous system needs to be in this relaxed state for the optimal digestive cascade to occur. It is in this optimal parasympathetic state that the pancreas releases digestive enzymes and the gallbladder releases bile to emulsify and break down fat.

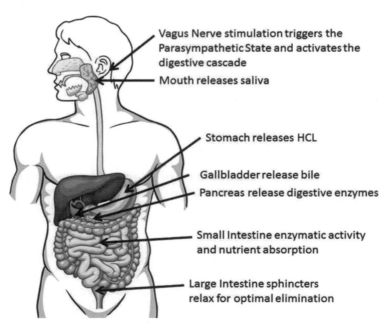

Vagus Nerve stimulation triggers the Parasympathetic State and activates the digestive cascade

Mouth releases saliva

Stomach releases HCL

Gallbladder release bile
Pancreas release digestive enzymes

Small Intestine enzymatic activity and nutrient absorption

Large Intestine sphincters relax for optimal elimination

Indications of Poor Digestion

- ❑ Eating meals under stress or on the run
- ❑ Dry mouth
- ❑ Belching or gas within one hour after eating
- ❑ Heartburn or acid reflux, GERD
- ❑ Feeling bloated within one hour after eating
- ❑ Loss of taste for meat
- ❑ Undigested food in stool
- ❑ Constipation
- ❑ Stomach pains or cramps

To ensure optimal digestion in the parasympathetic state, you can apply the Vibrant Blue **PARASYMPATHETIC**™ blend to the vagal nerve (behind the earlobe and up one inch on the mastoid bone) before meals to stimulate the parasympathetic nervous system "rest-and-digest" state. This state supports:

- ➤ Release of saliva
- ➤ Stomach production of HCL
- ➤ Pancreatic release of digestive enzymes
- ➤ Gallbladder release of bile
- ➤ Small Intestine enzymatic activity and nutrient absorption
- ➤ Sphincters relaxation for optimal elimination

Releasing Digestive Enzymes

The pancreas secretes digestive enzymes that help break down the carbohydrates, proteins, and fats in food so the nutrients can be properly absorbed in the small intestine. The pancreas also controls blood sugar levels. If it is overworked and becomes fatigued, the pancreas may not make enough enzymes to break down food so the body can absorb nutrients adequately. Pancreatic enzymes speed up the necessary chemical reactions in your body to break down food. If the pancreas isn't releasing proper enzymes, you don't get the nutrition you need, because your body can't absorb fats and some vitamins and minerals from foods. You might also lose weight and experience other problems because your body doesn't absorb enough nutrients. For instance, tests may show your body is not receiving enough vitamin D despite adequate supplementation.

Symptoms of Poor Digestive Enzyme Function

- ❑ Pain or tenderness in your belly
- ❑ Bad-smelling bowel movements
- ❑ Diarrhea
- ❑ Gas
- ❑ Feeling full
- ❑ Fingernails chip, peel, break, or don't grow
- ❑ Tests reveal low levels of vitamin D or other minerals despite supplementation

To put the pancreas in balance, consider rubbing some **PANCREAS**™ on the fifth rib, 2 ribs down from the under the breast bone (where the underwire of a bra would hit) on the left side of the body to restore the pancreas to balance for optimal function.

Supporting Fat Digestion

As you may know, a critical component of fat digestion is bile, a yellowish-green fluid that is produced in the liver and stored and concentrated in the gallbladder. When we eat a meal that contains fat, the gallbladder secretes bile into the small intestine, where it helps emulsify the fat for digestion.

Bile also serves as a depository to carry toxins and old hormones out of the body. Ideally, the gallbladder releases bile into the small intestine where it breaks down the fat for the body to absorb, before being eliminated from the body in the stool. When we eliminate the bile, we eliminate the toxins along with it. Unfortunately, stress, hormones, and excess fat consumption can make the bile thick, viscous, and stagnant, which impedes its ability to flow both to the small intestine and out of the body. This results in the following problems:

> Fats and their corresponding fat-soluble vitamins A, D, E and K are not properly emulsified, digested, or absorbed. This robs the body of the building blocks it needs to create hormones and cells.
> Undigested fats rancidify, creating an additional toxic burden for the body.
> Toxins, waste, and old hormones that were stored in the bile for elimination via the intestines do not exit the body and are therefore reabsorbed, further adding to the body's toxic burden and contributing to hormonal imbalances and gallbladder challenges.

In other words, the good things can't get into the body and the bad things are not removed from the body.

Organs of Fat Digestion

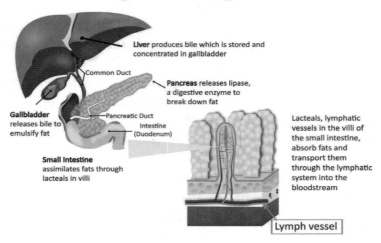

Liver produces bile which is stored and concentrated in gallbladder

Common Duct

Pancreas releases lipase, a digestive enzyme to break down fat

Gallbladder releases bile to emulsify fat

Pancreatic Duct

Intestine (Duodenum)

Small Intestine assimilates fats through lacteals in villi

Lacteals, lymphatic vessels in the villi of the small intestine, absorb fats and transport them through the lymphatic system into the bloodstream

Lymph vessel

Symptoms of Poor Fat Digestion

- ❏ Dry skin and brittle hair
- ❏ Hormonal imbalances (fat helps synthesize new hormones and eliminate old hormones)
- ❏ Low levels of fat-soluble vitamins like A, D, E, and K despite ample supplementation
- ❏ Gas, belching, or bloating after meals
- ❏ Mild headaches over the eyes
- ❏ Greasy, smelly, light-colored and floating stools.
- ❏ Gallbladder pain (right side, under ribs), pain between the shoulder blades or gallstones
- ❏ Nausea or diarrhea after eating

Essential Oils to Support Fat Digestion

To ensure optimal fat digestion, you might consider the following essential oils:

Liver: The liver produces bile, a yellowish-green fluid that aids in the emulsification of fats and the digestion and absorption of fat-soluble substances, like vitamins A, D, E, and K. The liver also stores fat-soluble toxins, including old hormones (like excess estrogen), in the bile for transport out of the body through the digestive elimination process. This means the liver needs to be functioning optimally to both produce bile and filter and store old hormones. You can support optimal liver function by applying Vibrant Blue Oils LIVER™ over the liver (right side of the body, under the ribs) 2 to 3 times daily.

Gallbladder: Once the liver produces bile, it is stored and concentrated in the gallbladder. When we eat a meal with fat, the bile should flow freely into the small intestine to break down the fat so we can absorb it. Unfortunately, stress, hormones, and excess fat consumption can make the bile thick, viscous, and stagnant, which impedes its ability to flow. Vibrant Blue Oils GALLBLADDER™ can help ease bile flow for optimal fat assimilation and absorption. To support the optimal flow of bile from the gallbladder, apply it on the right side of the body under the bra underwire or along and slightly under the right rib cage.

Lymph: After dietary fat is emulsified by bile and broken down by pancreatic lipase enzymes, the lymphatic system assimilates and absorbs the fat and fat-soluble vitamins into the bloodstream. Tiny lymphatic vessels in the villi of the small intestine, known as lacteals, absorb digested fats and transport these fats through the lymphatic system into the bloodstream for circulation throughout the body. LYMPH™ applied over the small intestine can help with the assimilation and transport of fat and fat soluble vitamins.

Intestinal Support

The intestines run from the stomach to the anus. The job of the small and the large intestines is to absorb nutrients and water and convert the waste to be expelled from the body through defecation. This absorptive quality makes the intestines prone to accumulating toxins and pathogens, passing them into the body in instances of increased intestinal permeability and constipation.

The Vibrant Blue Oils **PARASYMPATHETIC**™ oil blend optimizes motility and intestinal support. Additional essential oils for the intestines are discussed more thoroughly in Chapter 8.

General Digestive Discomfort

For symptoms of upset stomach, indigestion, food poisoning, or eliminating parasites, Vibrant Blue Oils **DIGEST**™ blend, inhaled or applied over the stomach area either directly or with a hot, wet compress, can bring relief to symptoms of discomfort.

Similarly, Vibrant Blue Oils **NERVE REPAIR**™ and **ANTI-INFLAMMATORY**™ help relieve pain, fight infection, and ease inflammation. Apply both directly over the area of discomfort. They can be used together or individually.

Chapter 8

Gut Repair and Inflammation

D isease begins in the gut because it is the main doorway into the body. It is the channel for healing nutrients to be absorbed and pathogens to be blocked. If this doorway isn't working properly, the health-promoting nutrients the body needs to heal are not well-assimilated, and harmful toxins can enter.

The epithelial cells lining the small intestine are connected by semi-permeable, tight junctions that serve as important gatekeepers. These tight junctions block the bad guys—undigested food, bacteria, fungus, yeast, parasites, and other toxins—while the microvilli on the tips of the epithelial cells selectively assimilate and absorb the good guys, the vital nutrients the body needs.

When digestion works optimally, the tight junctions stay closed, selectively screening all organisms and letting only nutrients pass into the blood stream. Like a good goalie on a soccer team, these tight junctions block unwanted microbes and toxins from entering the body, while selectively allowing nutrients to be absorbed. Now imagine that same soccer goal expanded to two to three times larger than its normal size. It would be a lot harder for the goalie to defend, right?

The same is true for defending against pathogens when the gut is inflamed. Gut inflammation from food allergies, stress, undigested food, toxic chemicals, parasites, or infections can compromise these tight junctions, leading to increased permeability and allowing harmful pathogens or undigested food to "leak" into the body. This triggers an inflammatory immune response where these toxins and undigested foods are tagged as "foreign invaders" and attacked by the body's immune system.

Intestinal inflammation also damages microvilli along the intestinal lining, impeding their ability to manufacture the digestive enzymes they need to break down the food for proper digestion, which prevents vital nutrients from being properly digested, absorbed, and assimilated and can lead to food allergies or intolerances.

undigested food particles and toxins

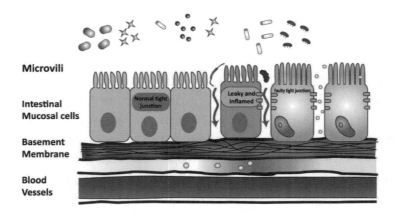

Inflammation in the gut can also drive chronic systemic inflammation elsewhere in the body, including the brain. The gut-brain axis is a two-way information channel: the brain sends signals to the gut, and the gut sends signals back to the brain. For example, 80 percent of the body's immune cells, known as Peyer's Patches, can be found in the lowest part of the small intestine, called the ileum. The Peyer's Patches should diffuse any threat from pathogens in the digestive track on site in the small intestine. But when the gut is leaky, toxins enter the bloodstream, triggering an inflammatory response. This gut-generated inflammation sends inflammatory signals to the brain, contributing to neuro-inflammation and degeneration. More specifically, systemic inflammation in the gut generates increased production of inflammatory proteins that alter brain neurochemistry and activate brain inflammation.

Similarly, larger compounds, not meant to be absorbed from the gut into the bloodstream, can leak from the gut into the blood, enter the brain, trigger an immune response, and set off systemic inflammation.

Finally, researchers have found that gut flora influence not only gut chemistry but also brain chemistry, including depression. Serotonin, the "feel-good" neurotransmitter, contributes to a sense of well-being. The gut hosts more than 90 percent of the body's serotonin! Remember our discussion of the vagus nerve and its connection between the brain and the gut? Researchers believe this connection influences mood. For example, people with irritable bowel syndrome also are prone to depression and anxiety.

Heal the Gut to Heal Systemic Inflammation

Inflammation is the body's attempt to protect and heal itself. Acute inflammation is good. Chronic inflammation is not. Chronic inflammation can last for years. When it isn't regulated, inflammation can lead to serious health conditions, including autoimmunity, food intolerances, anxiety, depression, poor focus and concentration, digestive dysfunction, high blood pressure, fluid retention, asthma, dementia, cramps, and ADD/ADHD.

In fact, doctors and alternative health practitioners consider inflammation to be the most important indicator for overall health. Reduce inflammation and, often, everything else falls into place.

Inflammation begins in the gut and spreads through the body. Therefore, if you can heal inflammation at its root—in the gut— you can protect the rest of the body.

All of the issues below are caused by systemic inflammation (with an inflamed gut as the cause):

- ❑ Digestive complaints such as gas, bloating, acid reflux, constipation, diarrhea, or irritable bowel syndrome (IBS)
- ❑ Seasonal allergies, sinus infections, or asthma
- ❑ Brain complaints like brain fog, chronic headaches, depression, anxiety, ADD/ADHD
- ❑ Hormonal imbalances such as PMS or PCOS
- ❑ Autoimmune diseases such as rheumatoid arthritis, Hashimoto's thyroiditis, lupus, psoriasis, or celiac disease.
- ❑ Low energy or fatigue
- ❑ Skin complaints: itchy skin, rashes, eczema, rosacea, acne, and hives
- ❑ Joint pain, muscle pain, headaches, or arthritis
- ❑ Candida overgrowth or strong cravings for sugar or carbohydrates
- ❑ Food intolerances, sensitivities, or allergies
- ❑ Nutritional deficiencies

This chronic inflammation and immune response cycle, left unchecked over time, can lead to autoimmune issues. Often, when inflammation becomes chronic, no discernible symptoms present until there is a loss of function.

How the Gut Triggers Systemic Inflammation

I had long wondered how inflammation that originates in the gut could impact the brain, and other areas of the body.

Paleomom.com's Sarah Ballantyne clearly explains this in her book *The Paleo Approach: Reverse Autoimmune Disease and Heal Your Body*, noting, "the pro-inflammatory and anti-inflammatory signals sent by cytokines, when produced in substantial quantities as occurs in anyone with leaky gut , travel throughout the body (via the blood) and transmit their message to virtually every cell, including cells in the brain." These signals can cross the blood brain barrier and activate an inflammatory response in the brain. "As inflammatory signals from the gut persist, the inflammation in the brain increases. An inflamed brain has less (and slower) nerve conduction, which manifests as mood related symptoms such as stress, depression, or anxiety," according to Ballantyne.

Ballantyne further notes that "once these inflammatory cells are activated in the brain, it can be hard to deactivate them, meaning that inflammation in the brain can be hard to turn off and inflammation in the brain will obstruct healing of the gut because of decreased vagus-nerve activation." She explains that many of the beneficial effects of the probiotic bacteria in the gut are dependent on the vagal activation affecting brain function (that occurs in the parasympathetic state). "Eighty percent of the fibers in the vagus nerve carry information from the gut to the brain and not the other way around. This means that the gut (and even the gut microflora) communicates directly with the brain, perhaps having a direct impact on emotions and moods," according to Ballantyne.

How to Heal the Gut

Healing the gut can reduce systemic inflammation. It requires a combination of dietary changes, select supplements, and essential oils. As everybody is different (I call this "bio-individual"), I encourage you to work directly with a healthcare practitioner to customize the suggested protocol to your specific needs.

Similarly, essential oils, like Brain Balance **ANTI-INFLAMMATORY**™ can be topically applied to regions of the brain to help turn off brain inflammation so the gut and the body can communicate and heal.

Support Optimal Digestion

For healing to begin, the body needs to be in the healing parasympathetic state. It is only in this state where the optimal digestive cascade can occur. Attempting to consume healing nutrients under stress in the sympathetic state will lead to impaired digestion that will further contribute to inflammation.

The critical first step to healing the gut is to eat in the optimal "rest-and-digest" parasympathetic state. You can do this by taking the time to sit down, relax, and breathe before eating. I also recommend applying a drop of **PARASYMPATHETIC**™ oil to the vagus nerve (behind the earlobe and up one inch on the mastoid bone) before meals to trigger optimal digestion.

Stimulating the parasympathetic state routes increased blood flow to the small intestine, allowing for healing of the intestinal wall and optimal enzymatic activity and nutrient assimilation. The parasympathetic state also triggers peristalsis, the muscle contractions that move food and waste through the digestive tract. If motility is impaired, the inability to move food through the intestines leads to abnormal fermentation, intestinal bacteria, yeast overgrowth, or unhealthy digestive conditions such as irritable bowel syndrome and small intestine bacterial overgrowth (SIBO).

Reduce Inflammation

For the gut to heal, you need to remove the source of damage, which could include chronic stress, the consumption of inflammatory foods—including too much sugar or foods you are sensitive to—medications, dehydration, alcohol, or intestinal infections (like candida, parasites, and SIBO). Consider a strict elimination diet that removes all grains, sugar, dairy, corn, soy, and in some cases nuts, eggs, and nightshades.

You also need to stop the inflammatory cascade to give the intestines the opportunity to heal. A good friend likes to say that you can't mow the lawn when the house is on fire. So long as the fire of inflammation is burning inside the gut, the body is going to invest resources in fighting the fire, not cleaning up the damage from the fire.

So how do we fight a fire in the intestines when they are inflamed and cannot assimilate nutrients? This is where the backdoors of topical application of essential oils and the olfactory channel work such magic.

Topically applied or inhaled essential oils can target and support the reduction of inflammation in the gut, even when the digestive channel is blocked.

Modulate the Histamine Response

To put out the fire of inflammation, we need first to modulate the immediate inflammatory response of histamine.

Histamine is a chemical neurotransmitter released at the mucosal surfaces in response to injury and allergic or inflammatory reactions. Histamine causes blood vessels to dilate and smooth muscle to contract, so the capillaries become more permeable to white blood cells, which can then quickly find and attack the infection or problem.

The increased permeability of the capillaries causes fluid to move out of capillaries, which gives rise to the classic symptoms of allergy such as a runny nose, watery eyes, and other noticeable symptoms in the gut, throat, lungs, skin, brain, and the entire cardiovascular system. Histamine also regulates physiological function in the gut and acts as a neurotransmitter in the brain.

While the release of histamine is a normal defense mechanism, an exaggerated histamine response can bind to cell receptor sites, causing irritation and chronic inflammation. This inflammation of the nasal passages, sinuses, lungs, and eyelids can cause sneezing; a runny nose; watery, red, itchy eyes; rashes; and breathing troubles such as wheezing, severe coughs, asthma, or hiccups. Inflammation of the small intestine can present as food allergies and sensitivities. Inflammation of the brain presents as fatigue, headaches, and brain fog. Overactive histamine receptor cells trigger these immune system reactions.

Two enzymes break down excess histamine and prevent allergic reactions keep histamine levels in balance. One of these enzymes lives in the lining of our intestines and must be present to maintain balanced histamine levels in the gut. A damaged gut lining compromises the production and secretion of this enzyme allowing histamine to build up and wreak havoc throughout the body.

Histamine Response

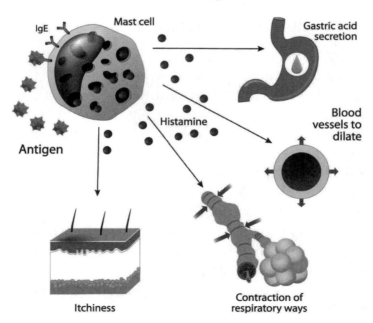

Symptoms of Histamine Imbalance:

- ❑ Nasal congestion, runny nose, seasonal allergies
- ❑ Irritated, watery, or red eyes
- ❑ Itchy skin, eyes, ears, or nose
- ❑ Exaggerated response to bug bites or bee stings
- ❑ Tissue swelling or "throat tightening"
- ❑ Chest pain, racing heart, or a drop in blood pressure
- ❑ Anxiety or panic attack
- ❑ If lightly scratch stomach three times, red lines appear
- ❑ Fatigue, confusion, irritability
- ❑ Digestive upset, especially heartburn, indigestion, and reflux

The goal is to balance, not block, the histamine response because histamine performs critical functions in the body, contributing to hydrochloric acid production and neurotransmitter signals.

Essential Oils to Balance Histamine

HISTAMINE BALANCE™ helps reduce overactive histamine reactions and modulate the immune response. The essential oils in the blend are uniquely suited to modulate excess histamine excretion, balancing histamine levels and helping to reset the immune response and reduce allergic reactions. Blue Tansy, in particular, is known for neutralizing histamine and helping to control allergic reactions. For allergic reactions, smell or apply one or two drops behind your ears, on the back of your neck, or on your sternum to open airways. For the gut and food intolerance support, apply in a clockwise direction around the belly button. For brain congestion, apply one or two drops at the base of skull on the back of the head or the bottoms of the feet.

How to Reduce Inflammation with Essential Oils

Inflammation is a natural defense mechanism designed to protect the body from infection and injury and repair damaged tissue. It allows for an increase in blood flow, bringing fluid, proteins, and white blood cells to the damaged tissue so it can heal. The increased blood supply results in redness, swelling and heat. Pain and immobility also protect the area and facilitate healing.

A prolonged inflammation and immune response cycle, when left unchecked over time in the gut, can spread elsewhere in the body, contributing to health challenges including:

➤ Digestive issues such as gas, bloating, diarrhea, or irritable bowel syndrome.
➤ Seasonal allergies, sinus infections, or asthma
➤ Hormonal imbalances such as premenstrual syndrome or polycystic ovary syndrome.
➤ Autoimmune diseases such as rheumatoid arthritis, Hashimoto's thyroiditis, lupus, psoriasis, or celiac disease
➤ Chronic fatigue or fibromyalgia
➤ Mood and mind issues such as depression, anxiety, ADD, or ADHD
➤ Skin issues such as acne, rosacea, or eczema
➤ Achy joints, headaches, arthritis
➤ Candida overgrowth or strong cravings for sugar or carbohydrates
➤ Food allergies or food intolerances

Inflammation is also an immune response that causes even more stress on your system. If your body is focused on fighting the war, it ignores the little battles like filtering out the blood, calming inflamed areas of the body, fighting bacteria, and regulating the gut, creating a tipping point to autoimmunity.

If you can heal inflammation at its root—in the gut—it may help with healing elsewhere in the body.

How to Heal Gut Inflammation

Removing inflammatory foods can help, but often not as quickly or efficiently as we would like, which would explain why people stay on elimination diets for months and sometimes years with little noticeable improvement. Imagine the impact of expediting the healing for the inflammatory process.

Topical application of ANTI-INFLAMMATORY™ rubbed clockwise around the belly button two or three times daily helps to reduce inflammation and encourage regeneration of chronically inflamed, damaged tissues. ANTI-INFLAMMATORY™ can also be topically applied to regions of the brain (behind the ear on the mastoid bone) or lightly around the base of the skull to help turn off brain inflammation so the gut and the body can heal.

Repair Intestinal Mucosal Lining

Healthy gut flora and a healthy mucosal lining are critical for absorbing nutrients from food and neutralizing toxic substances.

The intestines are lined with a thick bacterial band attached to the gut mucosal lining that plays host to our gut flora, helping to keep it healthy and intact. In her book, *Gut and Psychology Syndrome*, Dr. Natasha Campbell-McBride notes, "healthy indigenous gut flora has a good ability to neutralize toxic substances, inactivate histamine, chelate heavy metals, and other poisons. The cell walls of the beneficial bacteria absorb many carcinogenic substances, making them inactive. They also suppress hyperplastic processes in the gut, which is the basis of all cancer formation." In other words, if the intestinal mucosa nourishes the gut flora to keep it healthy and working properly, it neutralizes all other health threats.

Healthy intestinal mucosa is the glue that helps the gut flora, or the probiotics that feed the flora, stick to the gut lining. If the ability of the mucosal lining to protect the intestinal walls against pathogens and damage from food and waste is diminished, the beneficial effects of a nutrient-dense diet and probiotics are also diminished. It is like trying to apply wallpaper without glue. It will not stick where you want it to go.

Not only does the gut lining serve as a physical barrier and the first line of defense between the body and any pathogens we might swallow, but healthy gut flora helps us process and eliminate toxins and reduce inflammation, so maintaining its integrity is of the utmost importance.

Symptoms of Damaged Intestinal Mucosa

- ❑ GI sensitivity (cramps, diarrhea/constipation)
- ❑ Bloating or foul-smelling gas
- ❑ Persistent flatulence, burping, bloating
- ❑ Dysbiosis, including IBS or partially digested stools
- ❑ Yeast infections, thrush, cold sores, diaper rash
- ❑ Headaches, migraines, joint aches
- ❑ Food intolerances
- ❑ Leaky gut
- ❑ Chronic pain and fatigue
- ❑ Autoimmune conditions

Essential Oils to Repair the Mucosal Lining

To help balance and heal the intestinal mucosal lining, apply Vibrant Blue Oils **INTESTINAL MUCOSA**™ blend in a clockwise direction around the belly button two to three times daily. This helps restore the integrity of the mucosal lining to restore an optimal balance of healthy intestinal flora.

This essential oil blend is the missing link that allows all of our nutrient-dense whole food efforts and aggressive supplementation to absorb and assimilate so that healing can begin. And once the integrity of the intestinal mucosal wall has been re-established, the small intestine can do its job neutralizing the histamines and other toxins, in essence preventing allergies, inflammation, and other immune responses.

Heal Infections by Fortifying Boundaries

Neutralizing gut infections like yeast, candida, parasites, and fungus can help reduce gut inflammation. Most nutrient and water absorption occur in the intestines. Due to their absorptive nature, the intestines are also an area where pathogens and infections can live and assimilate into the body, especially in instances of weak energetic boundaries.

Dysbiosis from Crohn's disease, celiac disease, irritable bowel syndrome (IBS), small intestinal bacterial overgrowth (SIBO), parasites, or excessive bacteria in the small intestine can be indicative of poor energetic boundaries.

When proper boundaries are in place, the bacteria in the colon help to digest foods and absorb essential nutrients. When boundaries are not clear, bacterial overgrowth invades your boundaries, interfering with the healthy digestive and absorption process.

The bacteria invade and take over the small intestine, leading to poor nutrient absorption or malabsorption of nutrients, particularly fat-soluble vitamins and iron. In some cases, the pathogens consume some of the nutrients, leading to unpleasant symptoms, including gas, bloating, and pain.

When you improve energetic boundaries, pathogens are no longer an energetic match and often dissipate, restoring the balance of healthy gut flora. This healthy balance of bacteria in the intestines helps to support the immune functions in the epithelial cells, like maintaining physical and chemical barriers and making the gut more acidic and hostile to invading bacteria.

Healthy flora also compete with potential pathogens for space and food. If your healthy gut bacteria are already using all the resources available, there's nothing left to feed the bad guys. They also help to modulate the inflammatory immune response and neutralize toxic substances.

Essential oils are a great tool for balancing gut flora. Unlike antibiotics, which attack bacteria indiscriminately, killing both the good and the bad, essential oils only attack the harmful bacteria, allowing our body's friendly flora to flourish.

Symptoms of Poor Intestinal Boundaries

- ❑ Bloating or swelling
- ❑ Abdominal cramps or pain
- ❑ Constipation or diarrhea
- ❑ A diagnosis of SIBO, Crohn's, or IBS
- ❑ Candida
- ❑ Parasites
- ❑ Nutrient malabsorption

Small Intestine Support

The small intestine upholds physical boundaries and plays a discerning role with emotions. In the digestion process, the small intestine absorbs and assimilates key nutrients while preventing harmful pathogens and toxins from entering the body.

On an emotional level, the small intestine plays a similarly discerning role with emotions, helping to understand experiences and determine healthy and appropriate relationships and boundaries. It is also an area where we can hold deep childhood scars of rejection, abandonment, or abuse; negative thoughts fueled by feelings of lack of self-worth, low self-esteem, loneliness, neglect, and anxieties about survival and success.

Vibrant Blue Oils Emotion Balance SMALL INTESTINE SUPPORT™ blend supports the healthy functioning of the small intestine as it sorts and transforms food, feelings, and ideas into useful ingredients for the body/mind. It also helps correct imbalances where you are overly in tune with other's feelings at the expense of your own.

Applying 2 to 3 drops around the belly button, the ears, and over the forehead and heart may help foster clear boundaries that are supportive and nurturing to your physical, emotional, mental, and spiritual health.

DIGEST™ is also supportive for eliminating parasites and easing general symptoms of upset stomach, indigestion or food poisoning. It can be inhaled or applied over the stomach area either directly or with a hot wet towel compress can bring relief to symptoms of discomfort.

Large Intestine Support

The large intestine lets go of those things that don't serve us. Physically, it lets go of waste after our upper digestive system has taken all the necessary nutrients out of the food we eat. Emotionally, it allows us to let go of patterns of negative thinking, destructive emotions, and spiritual blockages that prevent us from being our best.

Compromised large intestine energy presents as having a hard time moving on from difficult situations, or holding onto emotions that harm or fail to serve us. This holding on can manifest as an unwillingness to share emotions or be open with others—the phenomenon of "bottling up" emotions for years very often leads to chronic constipation.

To help the body let go, apply 2 to 3 drops of **LARGE INTESTINE SUPPORT**™ over the large intestine, around the ears, or on the forehead or the bottoms of the feet to help release past hurts and stuck or hidden negative emotions.

Chapter 9

Detoxification

Detoxification is a process to clear the body of toxins or other materials that cause adverse health effects. Your body naturally works to neutralize, transform, and release unwanted materials or toxins, but sometimes it cannot keep up with the quantity of toxins to be cleared. When the body cannot clear toxins, it stores them in safe places. For example, toxins may be stored in body fat, and yeast overgrowth in the intestines often shields the body from heavy metals.

To maintain a state of health, the body needs to catch up, rest, repair, and heal to clear out stored toxins, potential illnesses, and disease. Detoxification support can help eliminate toxins and support the body's detoxification and elimination systems.

Topically applied essential oils can support the organs of detoxification, including the liver, gallbladder, intestinal tract, kidneys, lungs, lymphatic system, and the skin. By supporting, improving, and optimizing the function of these organs of elimination, the body can metabolize and excrete the toxins.

A detox gives the digestive system, including the liver, a break by eliminating foods that are high in toxins or difficult for the liver to digest, absorb, and assimilate (think sugar, caffeine, and processed food). Once the liver has more energy freed up, it can then start on the work of housecleaning (i.e. cleaning out the toxins that have been stored in fat cells).

When most people hear the word "toxin," they think of heavy metals or pollution. But a toxin can be any substance that creates an irritating or harmful effect in the body, including undigested food (think fats or proteins), excess hormones (like estrogen), and yeast overgrowth or other digestive concerns. Toxins can limit the ability of cells to function, so the body safely stores them away to avoid any harm.

Symptoms of Toxicity

The symptoms below indicate a high toxic burden that might be improved by supporting the organs of detoxification.

- ❑ Allergies
- ❑ Sluggish elimination
- ❑ Skin rashes or irritation
- ❑ Fatigue or lack of energy
- ❑ Mild depression, anxiety or mental confusion (including brain fog or memory loss)
- ❑ Puffy eyes or bags under the eyes
- ❑ Insomnia
- ❑ Nausea
- ❑ Kidney or liver problems
- ❑ Muscle stiffness or aches and pains
- ❑ Poor balance
- ❑ Difficulty losing weight
- ❑ Restlessness
- ❑ Dizziness
- ❑ Vision problems
- ❑ Headaches
- ❑ Weakened immune system or low-grade infection

Even if you have only mild symptoms, healthy detoxification and liver health are paramount for good digestion, a healthy metabolism, and proper thyroid function. So a pro-active detoxification can enhance your health and avoid fatigue and digestive sensitivity.

Organs of Detoxification

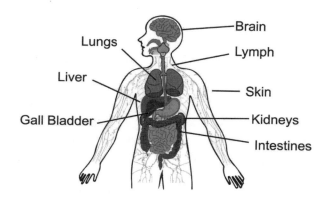

How can Essential Oils help with Detoxification?

The detoxification process mobilizes the toxins out of storage with the intent of then removing them from your body. Think of cleaning out your garage and putting all the trash in bags that you then take to the dump. Just as taking the garbage bags to the dump gets them out of your house, it is important that the toxins that are mobilized during the detoxification process leave the body. If they don't leave the body, they are recycled and reabsorbed (and sometimes into places that are not as safe as the fat cells, like the brain).

Popular detoxes do a terrific job of mobilizing the toxins, but unless the toxins leave the body, they can be reabsorbed and do more harm than they would have if just left alone. This is why it is important to include dietary fiber or clay in a detox effort: a binding agent moves the toxins out of the body. It is also important to support a detox with topically applied essential oils; they do not use an overburdened digestive system as a delivery channel to aid organ function and the elimination of toxins. Essential oils, with their ease of assimilation through the olfactory channel and the skin, are ideal tools to support detoxification of the body.

Drop into the Parasympathetic State

The autonomic nervous system has two states: the "fight-or-flight" sympathetic state and the "rest-and-digest" parasympathetic state. The parasympathetic state supports the body to detoxify and heal. You cannot heal when you are under stress. In addition to taking the time to relax, it is helpful to support the organs that oversee the body's stress, including the hypothalamus and adrenal glands. (See Chapter 5 on Stress for more.) Another key stressor and toxin creator is an impaired digestive system. If you are not absorbing and assimilating nutrients, it puts another stress on the body, and the undigested food particles add to the toxic burden.

To ensure optimal digestion, you can apply the PARASYMPATHETIC™ blend to the vagus nerve (behind the earlobe on the mastoid bone) before meals to stimulate the parasympathetic nervous system "rest-and-digest" state that promotes optimal digestion, absorption, and assimilation of the nutrients necessary to help the body heal and restore balance. For more information on the parasympathetic state, refer to Chapter 3.

Support the Liver

The liver is the primary organ of detoxification. It filters toxins and bacteria from blood and neutralizes the toxins in preparation for elimination. But dumping more toxins into an already overworked liver can be a recipe for disaster. The liver needs energy and vitality to keep up with the increased toxic burden.

Here's why. Detoxification should be part of the body's normal daily process. When we ate cleaner foods and lived in a cleaner environment, the body was probably able to keep up with the daily toxic burden. But for many of us, the toxic burden makes it difficult for our body to keep up. So, it is important to give the digestive system, liver, and gallbladder a little break to catch up on the detoxification process. This means mobilizing the toxins stored in fatty tissue and escorting them out of the body so they are not reabsorbed.

As you may know, any kind of detoxification effort increases the burden on the detox organs, including the liver, gall bladder, kidneys, lymphatic system, lungs, and skin. This requires optimal function from these organs. If they are already stressed, releasing additional toxins will only cause greater damage.

Symptoms of Liver Fatigue

Some indications that the liver might be overburdened and need detoxification support include:

- ☐ Easily intoxicated, hung over, or sick when drinking wine
- ☐ Frequent use of over-the-counter, prescription, or recreational drugs
- ☐ Sensitivity to tobacco smoke and chemicals like fragrances, cleaning agents, exhaust fumes, or strong odors
- ☐ Hemorrhoids or varicose veins
- ☐ Chronic fatigue or fibromyalgia
- ☐ Overconsumption of fast food, processed food, or products that contain artificial sweeteners, like Nutrasweet (aspartame)

Essential Oils for the Liver

Vibrant Blue Oils **LIVER**™ helps support optimal health and vitality of the liver. This is a great blend to support a detox cleanse, any kind of digestive repair effort that would release extra toxins (like yeast die-off), or for anyone who demonstrates liver stress symptoms like sensitivity to smells (smoke, perfume, etc.) and or chemicals, or those who are easily intoxicated or hung over.

Apply 2 to 3 drops of **LIVER**™ directly over the liver (right side of the body, under the breast) two to three times daily. The blend is especially helpful when applied before sleep during a detoxification effort as so much of the liver's work occurs while we are sleeping.

Support the Gallbladder

As you may know, the gallbladder is a small, pear-shaped organ that stores and concentrates bile, a yellowish-green fluid that is produced in the liver and stored and concentrated in the gallbladder. When we eat a meal that contains fat, the gallbladder secretes bile into the small intestine where it helps emulsify the fat for digestion.

Bile also serves to carry toxins and old hormones out of the body. Ideally, the gallbladder releases bile into the small intestine where it breaks down the fat for the body to absorb, before being eliminated from the body in the stool. When we eliminate the bile, we eliminate toxins with it.

Bile flows from the liver (releasing toxins with it) through the gallbladder to the small intestine, acting as a natural irritant to the lining of the intestine, which stimulates peristalsis that promotes bowel movements. This is one reason that poor gallbladder function and impeded bile flow contribute to constipation.

Unfortunately, stress, toxicity, hormones, or diets too low or too high in fat can make the bile thick, viscous, and stagnant, which impedes its ability to flow both to the small intestine and out of the body. This results in the following problems:

➤ Fats and their corresponding fat-soluble vitamins A, D, E, and K are not properly emulsified, digested, or absorbed. This robs the body of the building blocks it needs to create healthy hormones and cells.

➤ Undigested fats rancidify, creating an additional toxic burden for the body.

➤ Toxins, wastes, and old hormones that were stored in the bile for elimination via the intestines do not exit the body and are therefore reabsorbed, further adding to the body's toxic burden and contributing to hormonal imbalances and gallbladder challenges.

In other words, the good things can't get into the body and the bad things are not removed from the body.

Symptoms of Gallbladder Dysfunction

When there is not enough bile or bile is too viscous, it prevents us from properly digesting fats and can presents as symptoms like:

❑ Motion sickness
❑ Dry skin and brittle hair
❑ Constipation
❑ Hormonal imbalances (fat helps synthesize new hormones and eliminate old hormones)
❑ Low levels of fat-soluble vitamins like A, D, E, and K despite ample supplementation
❑ Gas, belching, or bloating after meals
❑ Mild headache above the eyes
❑ Greasy, smelly, light-colored, floating stools.

- Gallbladder pain (mid to right upper abdomen), pain between the shoulder blades or gallstones
- Floating stools, diarrhea, and greenish stools
- Hormone imbalances including premenstrual syndrome and menopause symptoms
- Gas, heartburn, and nausea after eating

Essential Oils for Gallbladder Support

Vibrant Blue Oils **GALLBLADDER**™ improves the viscosity of the bile to support the flow of bile and, with it, toxins out of the body. The gallbladder concentrates the bile to help break down fat and carry toxins out of the body. If the bile becomes too thick, it doesn't flow as well, and toxins don't move out of the system as efficiently.

To support the optimal flow of bile from the gallbladder, apply Vibrant Blue Oils **GALLBLADDER**™ on the right side of the body under the bra under-wire or along and slightly under the right rib cage two to three times daily.

Balance Estrogen

Estrogen serves as a stimulating hormone and plays many important roles in the body, ideally as part of a delicate balance with the calming hormone progesterone.

Estrogen dominance describes a hormonal imbalance between the levels of estrogen and progesterone. Estrogen dominance can throw off other functions in the body and contribute to weight gain, insomnia, infertility, impaired thyroid function, increased risk of cancer, and autoimmune disorders

Impaired detoxification can contribute to excess estrogen in the system. It requires a lot of effort and energy to eliminate estrogen from the body, and the liver plays a key role. If the liver is fatigued or overburdened with other toxins, estrogen can recirculate in the bloodstream. Estrogen is a long-acting hormone that will repeatedly deliver its chemical messages to the cells until it is successfully removed. Optimally, estrogen is also excreted in the feces. Some estrogen is packaged into bile, where it is excreted into the small intestines during digestion. There, the estrogen passes out of the body as part of solid waste. If there is constipation or slow transit time, the estrogen can be reabsorbed by the body and sent into recirculation.

Symptoms of Estrogen Dominance

When levels of the stimulating hormone estrogen fall out of balance with the calming hormone progesterone, the following symptoms can present:

- ❑ Anxiety, irritability, anger, agitation
- ❑ PMS, menstrual cramps, heavy or prolonged bleeding, clots
- ❑ Water retention/weight gain, bloating
- ❑ Breast tenderness, lumpiness, enlargement, fibrocystic breasts
- ❑ Mood swings, depression, weepiness
- ❑ Headaches/migraines
- ❑ Food cravings, sweet cravings, chocolate cravings
- ❑ Muscle pains, joint pains, back pain
- ❑ Foggy thinking, memory difficulties
- ❑ Fat gain, especially in abdomen, hips, and thighs
- ❑ Cold hands or feet
- ❑ Fatigue
- ❑ Trouble sleeping/insomnia
- ❑ Hair loss
- ❑ Thyroid dysfunction or sluggish metabolism
- ❑ Decreased libido/sex drive
- ❑ Allergic tendencies including asthma, rashes, acne or hives
- ❑ Gallbladder problems

Essential Oils for Estrogen Dominance

ESTROGEN BALANCE™ is designed to support the liver with the gentle mobilization of estrogen. Apply 2 to 3 drops over the liver with a castor oil pack three times weekly. You can also apply to the liver (right side of the body under ribcage) or on liver reflex points on the bottom of the right foot (beneath the ball of your foot from the pinky to the third toe). For optimal results, use the oil in combination with a binding agent such as chia seeds, flax seeds, hemp seed, charcoal, or psyllium.

Aid the Lymphatic System

Your lymphatic system removes waste from every cell in your body. It works as the body's septic system, removing the byproducts and wastes created from metabolizing nutrients. Just like the drains in your home, the lymphatic system can get congested and stagnant, and toxins can build up. The more you can help the lymph fluid flow, the more quickly you can move toxins out of the body.

Attempts to detoxify your body when the lymph system is congested often lead to detox and healing reactions. The lymphatic system aids the immune system in removing and destroying debris, dead blood cells, pathogens, toxins, excess fluid, and waste products from the cells and the interstitial spaces between the cells. It also absorbs fats and fat-soluble vitamins from the digestive system and delivers these nutrients to the cells of the body. Unlike the cardiovascular system, the lymphatic system does not have a central pump—it only moves as the muscles squeeze it along. So the lack of movement makes the lymphatic system stagnant, with waste accumulating and excessive toxins building up.

Symptoms of Sluggish Lymph Movement

If the lymphatic system is not working correctly, elimination, detoxification, and immunity may be affected, resulting in symptoms such as:

- ❑ Soreness and stiffness in the morning
- ❑ Fatigue or lack of mental clarity
- ❑ Bloating and water retention, rings get tight on fingers
- ❑ Dry or Itchy skin or a mild rash
- ❑ Congestion, stuffy head, sinus or periodontal infection
- ❑ Brain fog
- ❑ Cold or swollen hands and feet
- ❑ Weight gain, bloating around the abdomen, or cellulite
- ❑ Swollen glands, including breast tenderness

Major Causes of Lymphatic Congestion

➢ **Stress**—Stress-fighting hormones produce free radicals as waste products, which are highly acidic, altering our cellular chemistry and leading to poor drainage of the lymphatic system.

➢ **Digestive Imbalances**—Imbalanced gut flora can cause lymph congestion. A high concentration of lymph surrounds the gut; healthy gut flora are critical for proper lymph flow, detoxification, assimilation, and immunity.

➢ **Sedentary Lifestyle**—Lymph fluid is pumped through muscular contractions, so if you don't move your body, the lymphatic system will also eventually become inactive and will create toxicity in lymphatic-related tissues such as the breasts, skin, joints, and muscles.

➤ **Iodine Deficiency**—Iodine helps to mitigate the effects of a toxic environment and supports the lymph at the cellular level.

➤ **Dehydration**—Lymph is fluid, and the body needs to be hydrated to keep it flowing.

➤ **Imbalanced Diet**—Overconsumption of proteins and mucus-forming substances like milk, processed food, or sugar will also burden the lymph system, causing it to become congested and stagnant.

How to Get your Lymph Moving?

The top 3 ways to detoxify and cleanse your lymphatic system include:

1. Rebounding on a small, indoor trampoline
2. Dry brushing or sauna
3. Vibrant Blue Oils **LYMPH**™ blend also helps keep lymph flowing to move toxins out of the body. It can be used alone or in combination with other techniques to help increase circulation of fats and white blood cells within the lymphatic system for optimal delivery of nutrients to cells and removal of waste from the cells. We recommend liberally applying 2 to 3 drops each to the sides of the neck, the lymph nodes under the arms, and around inguinal ligament (bikini line area—think where your leg creases when you lift it) for a week before beginning a detox or healing protocol to ensure optimal drainage and health.

Skin

The sweat glands of the skin act as one of the body's avenues for elimination. When sweat passes through your sweat glands, it carries toxins out with it. The surface area of the skin covers 11,000 square feet, making sweating therapy effective to remove toxins. Supporting the detoxification pathway via the skin can lessen the burden on other organs like the liver and the kidneys.

For example, consider a detox bath with two cups of Epsom salt, one cup of baking soda, and a few drops of Vibrant Blue Oils **PARASYMPATHETIC**™ oil. The clove oil in the parasympathetic blend helps to pull toxins out of the skin to lessen the burden on the other organs of detoxification. For more detox bath recipes, visit http://www.vibrantblueoils.com/

Intestines

The intestines play an important role in detoxification. The small intestine shields the body from pathogens released during detoxification. The large intestine converts waste into stool to be expelled from the body through defecation. For more information on essential oils to support the intestines, go to Chapter 8.

Attend to Emotional Release

The detoxification process occurs on the physical, spiritual, and emotional levels and can help uncover and express feelings, especially hidden frustrations, anger, resentments, or fear. **Often, the more toxins a person releases, the more stored emotion that is also released.** It is important that you allow these emotions to be processed and released to avoid causing additional stress that would undermine the detoxification process.

Symptoms of Emotional Detoxification

When toxic emotions are present in the liver and gallbladder, they can present as symptoms like:

- ❑ Irritability or impatience
- ❑ Inappropriate anger, including angry outbursts or "flying off the handle"
- ❑ Over-reactivity or difficulty letting things go
- ❑ Feelings of not being heard, not experiencing love, not being recognized, inability to be honest with yourself or others
- ❑ Resentment, frustration, or bitterness
- ❑ Being judgmental, overly critical, fault-finding, or complaining
- ❑ Feeling the need to control situations or being domineering or bossy

Essential Oils for Detoxifying Emotions

Vibrant Blue Oils **LIVER SUPPORT**™ helps support the release of emotions, including frequent irritation, impatience, resentment or frustration, being critical of yourself or others, control issues, an inability to express your feelings, feelings of not feeling heard, not feeling loved, not being recognized or appreciated.

For more information on how essential oils can support emotions, refer to Chapter 6.

Support the Kidneys

The kidneys play a vital role in detoxification, regulating the flow and balance of fluids in the body, filtering the blood, and helping remove waste from the body through urination.

In Chinese medicine, the kidneys are considered the seat of courage and willpower. They control the volume, composition, and pressure of fluids in all the cells. Blood flows through the kidneys at its highest pressure, filtering out toxins and directing nourishing materials to where they are needed. Water is symbolic of the unconscious, emotion, and of that which we do not understand and that which we fear. Feelings of fear and paranoia can be held in the kidneys, impairing function.

Applying Vibrant Blue Oils **KIDNEY SUPPORT**™ over the kidneys (lower back, size of a fist starting at bottom rib), over the forehead or around the outside of earlobes can help you flow through fear and enhance the kidney's ability to release toxins.

Lungs

The lungs help energy flow in and out of the body, transporting oxygen from the atmosphere into the capillaries and releasing carbon dioxide (the waste gas resulting from breathing) from the bloodstream into the atmosphere. Feelings of grief, bereavement, regret, loss, and remorse can obstruct the ability of the lungs to accept and relinquish, impeding their function of "taking in" and "letting go." Grief that remains unresolved can become chronic and create disharmony in the lungs, weakening the lung's ability to flow oxygen through our system.

Apply Vibrant Blue Oils **LUNG SUPPORT**™ over the lungs to help flow through feelings of grief.

Similarly, **BREATHE**™ blend opens and soothes the physical airways to allow for enhanced oxygen intake and release. Formulated with three different types of eucalyptus essential oil that are known to increase blood flow by relaxing the blood vessels, thereby allowing more blood to circulate.

Both **BREATHE**™ and **LUNG SUPPORT**™ can be inhaled or topically applied over the lungs before yoga to optimize breath

BREATHE™ contains hot oils and should be diluted with another oil (like coconut oil or olive oil) prior to topical application. For more information on essential oils for respiration and circulation, see Chapter 10.

Purify the Air

To help neutralize environmental toxins like mold, consider diffusing **PURIFICATION™** or **HISTAMINE BALANCE™**.

Chapter 10

Brain Support: Blood Sugar and Circulation

Essential oils are ideal tools for supporting the brain as the olfactory channel carries them directly into the brain. They also can be topically applied to stimulate specific areas of the brain.

For example, using the **PARASYMPATHETIC**™ blend to stimulate the vagus nerve (behind the ear lobe on the mastoid bone) can both trigger the parasympathetic state and re-wire the brain to activate the parasympathetic state with every use.

Similarly, stimulatory oils, like two Vibrant Blue Oils Brain Balance blends, **FOCUS**™ and **ATTENTION**™, can be topically applied to specific areas of the head to stimulate and rewire neural pathways in specific regions of the brain, a concept known as neuroplasticity. Neuroplasticity is the brain's ability to adjust the activities of neurons in response to a change in the environment. Essential oils can facilitate just such a desired change.

It is important to note that neuroplasticity is not a one-size-fits-all magic bullet. It has tremendous benefit when used in very specific ways with proper dietary and nutritional support. Just as nutrition is highly bio-individual, the brain's rewiring in response to a change directed by an essential oil will be unique to each individual. Each brain is different, and what helps one person might hurt another. The information below is designed to help you use essential oils for brain rewiring to ensure positive, not negative, re-wiring.

Nourishing the Brain

As you may know, the brain needs three things:

1. Oxygen
2. Glucose
3. Stimulation

All three must be in place to build a healthy brain. I have been studying functional neurology with Datis Kharrazian, who literally wrote the book on brain health: *Why Isn't My Brain Working?*

According to Kharrazian, if you stimulate a brain that is deprived of oxygen or glucose, the additional stimulation will further fatigue the brain and cause damage. This is also true if you over-stimulate it beyond the point of fatigue, for example, if the brain starts to fatigue after 20 seconds and you continue stimulating beyond the point of fatigue, you are hurting the brain.

Just as you would never continue to run on a stress fracture as it would only cause further damage, stimulating an already fatigued brain beyond capacity will contribute to further faulty wiring, creating negative, not positive, neuroplasticity. This is one of the reasons that Dr. Kharrazian and his partner, acclaimed functional neurologist Brandon Brock, created an intense yearlong course to provide doctors with the clinical assessment tools to safely use the concepts of neuroplasticity on clients.

What is Neuroplasticity?

We know from the science of neuroplasticity that the brain creates communication pathways that help make recurrent thoughts and behaviors most efficient. The more we repeat a thought or activity, the more readily available those pathways become. For example, the more you practice a foreign language, musical instrument, or sport, the easier and more automatic the performance of that activity becomes. This is true for negative and positive thought patterns as well.

We can rewire the brain for positive neuroplasticity and reframe negative thought patterns, behaviors, and physiological responses. If we repeat negative thoughts and behaviors, like those related to anxiety, depression, worry, fear, anger, or grief, the brain will wire itself to make those negative neuroplasticity patterns more efficient.

Similarly, if we over-stimulate a brain that is deprived of oxygen and glucose and therefore too fatigued to receive new positive stimuli, negative neuroplasticity patterns can develop. It's a little bit like fueling exhausted adrenals with triple shots of espresso. You can stimulate the body and brain to function, but you will deplete the underlying adrenals even further. It holds true that networks that fire together wire together and faulty input creates faulty output.

A Bio-Individual Approach to Neuroplasticity

Just as you might approach nutritional support by looking at what the body needs, it is important to approach brain support in the same way. Protocols for impacting the brain should be customized for each individual based on the area and side of the brain that need stimulation and the duration of the stimulation based on when fatigue begins to set in.

It is important to assess and support the following areas before beginning any aggressive protocol to rewire the brain:

> Oxygen
> Glucose
> Stimulation

If an issue like pain or inflammation is affecting both sides of the body—for example, if you experience pain in both knees—it is likely that nutritional issues, including oxygen and glucose, are the underlying cause and must be addressed first. If you only experience an issue on one side of the body, then it often can be addressed by strengthening the corresponding area of the brain.

Essential Oils to Oxygenate the Brain

Healthy circulation is critical for delivery of oxygen and nutrient-rich blood to the body and the brain, while simultaneously carrying toxins and waste to the kidneys and liver to be eliminated.

An easy way to assess healthy circulation is to examine the circulation in distal regions like the fingers and the toes. The brain is also a distal region and as the most vertical tissue, it is consistently dealing with the forces of gravity due to its vertical position. One can assume that if circulation is poor in the distal regions of the fingers and toes, it is also poor in the brain.

Symptoms of poor circulation:

- ❑ No brain endurance for focus and concentration
- ❑ Cold hands, feet, and face
- ❑ Must exercise or drink coffee to improve brain function
- ❑ Poor nail health, white nail beds instead of pink
- ❑ Fungal growth on toenails
- ❑ The tip of the nose is cold
- ❑ Hair thinning or falling out

All of these indications reflect a lack of blood flow and nutrients to extremities. For example, blood flow to the scalp is responsible for carrying hormones and essential nutrients needed by the hair follicles. When circulation to the head is compromised, many individuals experience hair thinning and loss.

You can also compare the temperature of the fingers, the toes, and the nose to that of the arms and the legs or the rest of the face. The temperature will be the same as on the body if circulation is healthy.

If you notice poor blood flow to the extremities, you can assume that there is poor blood flow to the brain and any efforts to support neuroplasticity that lack appropriate oxygen and glucose will likely only fatigue the brain. The brain needs oxygen and glucose along with stimulation. Improving circulation will ensure that the brain has the raw materials it needs to build the neuroplasticity muscles with essential oil stimulation.

Brain Circulation

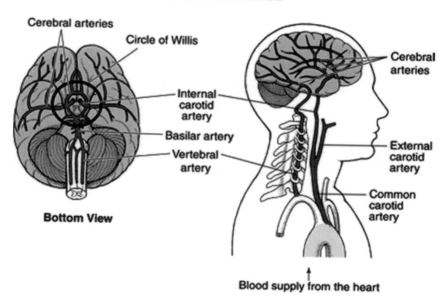

Essential Oils for Circulation:

The following essential oils can be used to stimulate blood flow in the veins and improve circulation:

CIRCULATION™: Formulated to help the circulatory system deliver oxygen and nutrients to every cell in the body and stabilize body temperature (especially in the extremities, like the fingers, toes and brain). Enhanced blood flow also helps maintain healthy PH levels, remove metabolic waste and protect against microbial and mechanical damage. To apply, massage 1 to 2 drops under the clavicle, behind the ears, on the wrists and ankles.

BREATHE™: Formulated with three different types of eucalyptus essential oil, which is known as a great vasodilator. As it enters the body, eucalyptus essential oil increases the blood flow by relaxing the blood vessels, thereby allowing more blood to circulate. **BREATHE™** can also help improve blood and oxygen flow to the brain. If poor circulation makes you feel tired or fatigued, apply 1 to 2 drops of **BREATHE™** over the heart and lungs.

HEART™: The heart integrates and balances the physical, emotional, and mental body, providing blood to every cell and every organ. The heart is also our body's reset button, but a state of constant stress can fatigue the heart and compromise our ability to reset, leading to inflammation, infections, toxicity, and heart disease. To return the heart to balance, support circulation, and balance blood pressure, apply 1 to 2 drops of **HEART™** over the heart.

ENERGIZE™: Formulated to improve circulation and restore the body's vitality and energy, **ENERGIZE™** contains several powerful oils like geranium to improve poor circulation by toning the blood vessels and peppermint to facilitate blood flow. To apply, massage 1 to 2 drops of **ENERGIZE™** over the heart.

LYMPH™: The lymphatic system works in tandem with the circulatory system. **LYMPH™** is uniquely formulated to increase circulation of fats and white blood cells within the lymphatic system for optimal delivery of nutrients to cells and removal of waste from the cells. To apply, massage 1 to 2 drops each to the sides of the neck, the lymph nodes under the arms, and around the inguinal ligament (bikini line area).

Peppermint is known to improve circulation, boost energy, and relax muscles. To apply, just smell or massage a drop or two over the heart.

Essential Oils for Optimal Brain Glucose

Glucose is fuel for the brain. The brain needs a constant steady supply of glucose (also known as blood sugar) at all times to function properly. Although the brain weighs only about two or three pounds, it uses about 30 percent of the body's total glucose.

Besides being the essential fuel source for neurons in the brain, glucose and insulin have significant impacts on amino acid transport across the blood-brain barrier, and proper glucose metabolism is critical for balanced neurochemistry. It is, therefore, important to keep glucose levels in the blood balanced and steady for optimal brain function.

Symptoms of Blood Sugar Imbalances:

❑ Cravings for sugar, carbohydrates, or coffee
❑ Sleepiness or energy dips in afternoon
❑ Irritability or feelings of shakiness if meals are skipped or delayed
❑ Difficulty concentrating when hungry
❑ Difficulty falling asleep or awakening hours after going to bed and finding it difficult to go back to sleep
❑ Fatigue after meals
❑ Weight in the abdomen or difficulty losing weight
❑ Frequent thirst or urination
❑ Need for stimulants such as coffee after meals

How Blood Sugar Works

Carbohydrates in the food we eat are digested and absorbed as glucose, then transported through the bloodstream, supplying energy to every cell in the body. The body is continually monitoring the levels of glucose (blood sugar) in the blood to ensure that it doesn't spike too high or dip too low. The goal is to maintain a condition of internal stability, which is necessary for optimal function.

Keeping blood sugar in balance is important for:

> Energy levels, including optimal sleep
> Brain health, including moods and mental focus.
> Hormonal balance
> Weight loss
> Optimal health, including the optimal function of every organ

Diet is a primary tool for controlling blood sugar, ideally limiting the intake of foods that spike blood sugar, like sugar and carbohydrates. Increasing the intake of healthy fats and supporting the body's ability to digest and assimilate fats can also help curb hunger cravings and sustain blood sugar levels for longer periods of time.

Essential oils to support the organs of blood sugar regulation:

PANCREAS™: The digestive system breaks down the carbohydrates from food into glucose, which goes straight into the bloodstream, causing blood sugar concentrations to rise. The pancreas releases insulin to transport the glucose into the cells. As more and more cells receive glucose, blood sugar levels return to normal. Excess glucose is stored as glycogen (stored glucose) in the liver and muscles. If you have not eaten for a while and blood glucose concentrations drop, the pancreas releases another hormone called glucagon. Glucagon triggers the breakdown of glycogen into glucose, thus pushing blood glucose levels back up to normal. **PANCREAS™** oil facilitates this normal function of the pancreas.

LIVER™: The liver acts as the body's glucose (energy) reservoir and helps to maintain steady and constant blood sugar levels by balancing the uptake, storage, and release of glucose, depending on the body's need for energy. More specifically, excess glucose is removed from the blood and converted into glycogen (the storage form of glucose), which is stored in the liver. When blood sugar levels drop, the liver initiates a process called glycogenolysis, where glycogen is converted back into glucose, or by converting other sugars into glucose, gradually releasing it into the bloodstream until levels approach normal range. Finally, the liver produces ketones from fats when glucose is in short supply.

ADRENAL™: Blood sugar imbalances can exhaust the adrenals. For example, eating a sugary meal will spike then quickly crash blood sugar, requiring the adrenals to release cortisol to stabilize blood sugar. Similarly, stress hormones such as adrenaline (epinephrine) can increase blood sugar levels to meet your body's demands for energy. Every stress response is a blood sugar response. Fatigued adrenal glands can struggle to produce and release cortisol, which in turn throws off the body's balance of blood sugar.

Essential Oils for Optimal Brain Stimulation

Vibrant Blue Oils Brain Balance blends **FOCUS™, BRAIN BOOST™, ANTI-INFLAMMATORY™,** and **ATTENTION™** can be used to provide gentle stimulation to specific regions of the brain to activate the neural pathways used in the processing of this stimulatory information.

Neuronal connections in these pathways are strengthened, and new connections are established through repeated sessions of multi-sensory input. This can include exercises like eye tracking and physical movement to stimulate that area of the brain.

Stimulation is often focused more heavily on one side of the body than the other, almost always on the weaker side. The goal is to strengthen the weaker side to return the body to balance. Strengthening the stronger side will throw off the imbalance even more.

This can be determined through a detailed checklist and a visit to a chiropractor trained in functional neurology, who can observe as you complete different physical tasks like rapidly rotating your hands at the same time to see which side of the body fatigues more quickly or balancing on one leg with eyes both open and closed. A trained professional will be able to identify:

1. The region of the brain that needs stimulating
2. The weaker side of the brain that needs strengthening to bring the entire brain back into balance
3. The point at which fatigue sets in and the stimulatory exercise should be discontinued.

This last point is critical. It is important to work with a trained professional to assess how much endurance you have for stimulating the brain. It is, unfortunately, common for people to fatigue the brain when they are attempting to rehabilitate the brain. They overdo it, the brain crashes, and their brain health regresses. Datis Kharrazian uses the example of rehabilitating a torn biceps by gently lifting some weights. "If you do it too aggressively, you're going to reinjure yourself. It's the same thing when you look at brain development issues, brain injuries, and neurodegenerative issues. You have to figure out what your endurance is."

A trained professional must guide you to learn how much stimulatory oil to apply and where to apply it. Some people can't handle direct activation, for example, if an area of the brain is too fatigued or too compromised from symptoms.

Where you apply brain-stimulating essential oils is important. Do not apply a stimulatory oil to an area of the brain that can be over-stimulated and more quickly fatigue the brain. For example, it is not advisable to apply stimulatory essential oils directly to the brain stem (the back center of the head, at the ridge where the neck meets the skull). I have found this application point is too intense for most clients. I originally looked at this point of application for the **PARASYMPATHETIC**™ blend as this is where the vagus nerve originates, but I realized that it also stimulates many other nerves in addition to the vagus nerve, opening the potential to overstimulate the brain and cause more damage.

A gentle application behind the ear lobe on the mastoid bone of the Vibrant Blue Oils **PARASYMPATHETIC**™ blend of clove and lime isolates and stimulates the vagus nerve in a very targeted and gentle way to avoid any harm. It is designed to gently drop the body into the parasympathetic state, which enhances the body's ability to balance and heal without impacting other areas of the brain, making it is safe to apply even if circulation and blood sugar are compromised.

Our other Brain Balance oils make excellent tools to facilitate neuroplasticity when used with the guidance of a trained professional. We are all different; a qualified practitioner can customize most treatments for the individual's specific needs and goals.

Chapter 11

Immune System

Essential oils provide key components of the plants' immune systems and protect plants from bacterial and viral infections. They work the same magic in us—preventing the onset of colds or nipping them in the bud. The blends below are some of my favorites for keeping my family healthy!

IMMUNE SUPPORT™

This blend traces its origins to the bubonic plague when thieves were stealing gold teeth out of the mouths of the dead. When they were apprehended, they were offered a lesser sentence in exchange for sharing how they avoided the illness. Their secret was this blend of hot oils that strengthen the immune system against flu, colds, and coughs as well as infections, viruses, bacteria, fungus, parasites, and microbes. To prevent illness or nip it in the bud once it starts, apply **IMMUNE SUPPORT™** 2 to 3 times daily on the throat (diluted) or to the bottoms of the feet. To keep your family healthy, rub the oil on the bottoms of the feet before bed. (Kids can even be asleep when you apply it.)

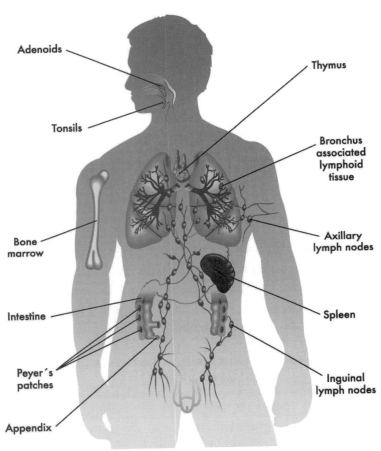

Organs of the Immune System

- Adenoids
- Thymus
- Tonsils
- Bronchus associated lymphoid tissue
- Bone marrow
- Axillary lymph nodes
- Intestine
- Spleen
- Peyer's patches
- Inguinal lymph nodes
- Appendix

THYMUS™

The thymus gland, located in front of the heart, plays an important role in the immune system, maturing infection-fighting white blood cells. Stimulating the thymus by gently tapping on the gland (thymus thumping) or using essential oils can increase the release of white blood cells. To stimulate immune function against infections, viruses, and bacteria, rub 2 to 3 drops of **THYMUS™** on the thymus (on the breastbone at the third rib) in a clockwise motion for 30 seconds, and then stimulate the thymus by gently tapping it.

SPLEEN™

The spleen, located in the left upper abdomen, is an important part of the immune system. It helps fight certain bacteria, like those that cause pneumonia and meningitis. It serves as a reservoir for blood, filtering and purifying the blood and lymph fluid that flow through it. A damaged spleen makes you more susceptible to infections. You can support the spleen by applying 2 to 3 drops of **SPLEEN SUPPORT**™ over the spleen (left side of the body, under the breast), over the forehead or around the earlobes.

LYMPH™

Your lymphatic system supports the immune response by bringing nutrients to the cells and helping to clear toxins from them. The lymphatic system is the body's first line of defense against disease. It includes lymph nodes (with clusters found in the neck, chest, underarms, abdomen, and groin). Unlike the cardiovascular system, the lymphatic system does not have a central pump—it only moves as the muscles squeeze it along. If the lymphatic system becomes stagnant, waste and excessive toxins accumulate, impacting immunity.

Lymph stagnation—when the fluid isn't flowing—can impede the body's ability to mount an immune response. To help increase circulation of white blood cells within the lymphatic system for optimal removal of waste from the cells, apply 2 to 3 drops of **LYMPH**™ to both sides of the neck, the lymph nodes under the arms, and around the inguinal ligament (the bikini line area, where your leg creases when you lift it). Promoting lymph flow around the neck can greatly relieve head congestion. The blend may be used liberally.

BREATHE™

BREATHE™ opens and soothes the airways and tissues of the respiratory system. It also reduces inflammation to support and relieve congestion, colds, flu, bronchitis, coughs, sore throats, sinus infections, pneumonia, and asthma. To apply, dilute with another oil, like castor oil, coconut oil, or olive oil and rub 1 to 2 drops topically on the throat and upper chest. You can also put a few drops on the pillowcase for respiratory conditions or apply a hot wet towel compress over the throat and keep it on for about 15 minutes. Put a few drops on the pillowcase at night. This oil can feel hot, so I do not recommend applying it undiluted to the skin.

HISTAMINE BALANCE™

Just smelling this blend can clear the sinuses or work magic on runny noses and allergies. HISTAMINE BALANCE™ contains Blue Tansy, which contains wonderful anti-inflammatory and anti-allergenic properties. For severe congestion or non-stop nasal drip and sneezing, apply a small amount to a cotton swab (make sure the cotton is tightly attached first). Then use the swab to coat the inside of each nostril gently. For acute nasal issues, insert it (gently!) high into the nasal canal and leave it for up to five minutes. This will often trigger the release of a lot of mucus followed by relief of symptoms. You also can rub it on the bottoms of the feet, behind the ears, or at the base of the neck to help relieve congestion, itchy eyes, and other cold, flu, or allergy symptoms. Repeat as needed throughout the day. It is also great for diffusing before bed.

SINUS SUPPORT™

This blend helps to clear and open the nasal passages and supports the relief of sinus pressure from chronic sinus infections and sinus issues related to allergies.

The sinuses are a connected system of hollow cavities in the skull that are lined with soft, pink tissue called mucosa. Normally, the sinuses are empty except for a thin layer of mucus. The sinuses drain into the nose through small holes. Sinusitis (or inflammation of the sinuses) can be uncomfortable and difficult to treat. The pockets become filled with thick mucus, bacteria, or fungus. The tissue swells, and the drainage openings into the nose become inflamed and blocked, no longer allowing fluid to escape. This then leads to the common symptoms of sinusitis: headaches, facial pressure, and even toothaches from surrounding nerve impingement.

Essentials oils can easily travel into the small holes to loosen mucus and promote drainage. Sinus Support works as a local decongestant, breaking up mucus, stimulating drainage of the nose and sinuses, and relieving head pressure. Essential oils are also antimicrobial, to help resolve infectious organisms such as bacteria, viruses, and fungus in the sinuses and nasal cavity.

Apply 2 to 3 drops of **SINUS SUPPORT™** to a cotton swab and swab the inside of the nasal passages 2 to 6 times daily. For optimal effectiveness, you can leave the swab in the nasal passage for up to 20 minutes. Try to relax and focus on breathing through the nose.

All of these oils can be added to a healing bath to boost the immune system and help your body release toxins more efficiently.

Appendix

Body Balance Blends

Proprietary body balance blends are formulated to balance key organs and systems of the body so the body can heal.

BLEND	INGREDIENTS	APPLICATION
Adrenal Balances adrenals to support anxiety, stress, low back pain and fatigue.	Galbanum, Thyme, Frankincense, Manuka and Rosemary.	Apply 1- 2 drops on the adrenal glands (lower mid-back, one fist above the 12th rib on each side) upon waking, before bed and throughout the day as needed.
Estrogen Balance Supports optimal liver function to gently mobilize and detoxify excess estrogen	German Chamomile, Orange, Rosemary, Celery Seed and Lemon.	Apply 2 – 3 drops over liver (right side of body under ribcage) or on liver reflex points on the bottom of foot (beneath ball of foot from pinky to 3rd toe).
Gall Bladder Supports viscosity of bile to support fat digestion, detoxification and constipation.	Black Cumin, Chamomile, Thyme and Rosewood.	Apply 2- 3 drops before meals underneath the ribs at the Gall Bladder (right side, under the third rib).
Heart Helps support cardio system and emotions associated with the heart.	Jasmine, Roman Chamomile, Spruce, Blue Tansy, Spikenard, Hyssop, Rose and Neroli.	Apply 1- 2 drops to heart as needed through the day.
Hormone Balance Supports the release of stored hormones and the fat they are stored in	rankincense, Holy Basil , Massoia Bark, Sage, Basil, Ylang Ylang and Geramium.	Apply 2- 3 drops to liver (right side of body under breast)
Intestinal Mucosa Helps revitalize healthy flora in the small intestine.	Cardamom, Nargarmotha, Birch Bark, Marjoram, Tarragon, Cypress and Elemi.	Apply 2- 3 drops in a clockwise circle around belly button, morning and night.
Liver Supports optimal liver health and function.	German Chamomile, Vitex Berry, Lemon, Balsam of Peru, Peppermint and Helichrysm.	Apply 2- 3 drops to liver (right side of body under breast) upon waking and before bed.
Lymph Supports optimal movement of lymphatic fluid throughout the body.	Palmarosa, Ylang Ylang, Spearmint, Helichrysm, Run Kewda and Vitex Berry.	Apply 2- 3 drops to lymph nodes (on neck, arm pits and groin) 2-3 times daily.
Pancreas Tonifies the pancreas, supporting healthy digestion and blood sugar handling.	Mhyrr, Patchuoli, Geranium, Anise Seed, and Rose Geranium.	Smell or apply 2- 3 drops to pancreas (2 ribs below breast on left side) before meals. Also smell before bed on a cotton ball inserted in a pillow case.
Thymus Strengthens the thymus gland for optimal immune support against infections, viruses, bacteria, fungus, parasites, tumors and inflammatio	Frankincense, Juniper Berry, Nutmeg, Holy Basil, Ravintsara, Rosemary, Oregano, Ginger, Blue Tansy, Black Cumin, Clove Bud and Hyssop.	Apply 2-3 drops on the thymus (breastbone at third rib) in a clockwise motion.

To learn more about specific oils included in each blend and how they work to support specific organs and regions of the brain, visit https://vibrantblueoils.com/bookbonus/

Brain Balance Blends

Proprietary brain balance blends are formulated to support optimal function of the brain to ensure that key hormonal and nervous system signals are sent and received.

BLEND	INGREDIENTS	APPLICATION
Anti-Inflammatory Supports pain and inflammation	Frankincense, Dill Seed, Cumin, Grapefruit, Rosewood, Ylang Ylang and Ginger.	Apply on vagal nerve (behind ear lobe on mastoid bone) or directly on area of inflammation
Attention Supports ADD and ADHD	Vetiver, Frankincense, Lavender and Cedarwood.	Apply 1- 2 drops on brain stem (back of the neck), temples, across the forehead and the bottom of the feet.
Brain Boost Supports extra thinking power	Ylang Ylang, Melissa, Sandalwood, Frankincense, Cedarwood, Lavender, and Helichrysum.	Apply on the back of the neck, temples, bottom of feet (big toe).
Circadian Rhythms Supports healthy circadian rhythms and sleep patterns.	Balsam of Peru, Grapefruit, Lavender, Rose Geranium, Myrtle, Myyrrh and Melaleuca.	Apply above ears, on top of skull and very back of the head before bed.
Circulation Supports healthy circulation to extremities	Cypress, Peppermint, Frankincense, Myrtle, Ginger, Black Pepper, Nutmeg, and Grapefruit	Apply 1- 2 drops under the collar bone, behind ears and at base of the skull. To warm extremities, apply on wrists and ankles.
Focus Supports mental alertness.	Rosemary, Basil, Holy Basil, Peppermint and Cardamom.	Apply across brow, back of neck, collar bone or on temples and wrists.
Histamine Balance Helps reduce over-active histamine reactions and modulate the immune response.	Blue tansy, Roman Chamomile, Vetiver, Peppermint, Rosemary, Lavender, Manuka, Ravensara and Spruce.	Apply 1 -2 drops on bottom of feet, at base of skull, behind ears, and sternum. Apply 1 - 2 drops to a Q-tip and gently swab inside both nostrils
Hypothalamus Supports the endocrine system	Frankincense, Bay Rum, Patchouli, Helichrysm, Sandalwood, Spruce and Red Mandarin.	Apply on forehead slightly above the third eye.
Parasympathetic Triggers the optimal rest and digest healing state.	Clove and Lime.	Apply on vagal nerve (behind ear lobe on mastoid bone).

To learn more about specific oils included in each blend and how they work to support specific organs and regions of the brain, visit https://vibrantblueoils.com/bookbonus/

Emotion Balance Blends

Proprietary emotion balance blends are formulated to acknowledge and release underlying emotions that can impede healing.

BLEND	INGREDIENTS	APPLICATION
Calm Supporting Anxiety	Tangerine, Orange, Ylang Ylang, Blue Tansy and Patchouli.	Apply over the heart, nape of the neck, wrists, on the forehead and outside of ears.
Bladder Support Releasing Trauma	Frankincense, Geranium, Helichrysum, Lavender, Petitgrain Combava, Rose, Sandalwood, Spruce and Valerian Root.	Apply over the bladder on the forehead or around the ears.
Kidney Support Releasing Fear	Cedarwood, Fir, Frankincense, Pine, Spruce and Ylang Ylang.	Apply over the kidneys (lower back), bottom of feet, on the forehead or around the ears.
Large Intestine Surrendering Control	Ylang Ylang Extra, Cedarwood, Frankincense, Rose, Elemi, Cinnamon, Cypress, Sandalwood, Helichrysum, Myrtle, Hyssop, Myrrh and Peppermint.	Apply over the large intestine and heart or on the forehead.
Liver Support Releasing Ange	Lavender, Geranium Bourbon, Elemi, Sandalwood, Blue Tansy, Ylang Ylang, German Chamomile, Cypress, Grapefruit and Helichrysum.	Apply over the liver (right side of body under breast) upon waking and before bed or as needed.
Lung Support Supporting Grief	Bergamot, Geranium, Lemon, Mandarin, Orange, Rose and Ylang Ylang.	Apply over the lungs and heart, around the ears or on the forehead.
Small Intestine Supporting Healthy Boundaries	Grapefruit, Lime, Litsea Cubeba, Mandarin, Sandalwood, Tangerine and Ylang Ylang Extra.	Apply over the belly button, around ears or in a bath.
Spleen Support Supporting Worry	Lavender, Vanilla and Patchouli.	Apply over the spleen (upper left abdomen) or on the forehead.
Thyroid Support Supporting Clear Expression	Angelica, Chamomile, Frankincense, Geranium, Hyssop, Lavender, Lemon, Myrrh, Neroli, Orange, Rose, Rosewood, Sage, Sandalwood, Spruce and Ylang Ylang.	Apply over the throat or around ears.
Uplift Supporting Depression	Ylang Ylang Rosewood, Spruce, Frankincense and Blue Tansy.	Apply on vagal nerve (behind ear, on neck). Can also apply over the forehead, the heart or areas of poor circulation.

To learn more about specific oils included in each blend and how they work to support specific organs and regions of the brain, visit https://vibrantblueoils.com/bookbonus/

Symptom Support Blends

Proprietary symptom support blends are formulated to support and relieve discomfort and painful symptoms while the underlying concerns are being addressed.

BLEND	INGREDIENTS	APPLICATION
Blood Sugar Balance Reduces hunger between meals and sugar and carbohydrate cravings	Grapefruit, Lemon, Peppermint, Cinnamon, Celery seed and Ginger.	Add 3 - 6 drops to water and drink between meals.
Breathe Supports the respiratory system.	Eucalyptus globulus, Eucalyptus citriodora, Myrtle, Eucalyptus radiata, Peppermint, Spruce, Ravensara, Pine and Marjoram.	Apply on throat and upper chest.
Digest Supports stomach upset.	Peppermint, Juniper, Anise, Fennel, Ginger root and Tarragon.	Apply over the stomach.
Immune Support Strengthens immune system and protects against flu, colds, coughs, infections, viruses and bacteria.	Cinnamon, Citronella, Clove, Eucalyptus, Ginger, Lemon, Mandarin, Mountain Savory, Nutmeg, Orange, Oregano, Rosemary and Thyme	Cinnamon, Citronella, Clove, Eucalyptus, Ginger, Lemon, Mandarin, Mountain Savory, Nutmeg, Orange, Oregano, Rosemary and Thyme Massage 2- 3 drops on feet twice daily. Dilute and apply on throat, around ears, on thymus and under the arms to strengthen the immune system.
Migraine Relief Offers relief from inflammation and associated migraine pain.	Basil, Marjoram, Lavender, Peppermint, Roman Chamomile, and Helichrysum.	Apply on forehead, temples and the back of the neck.
Nerve Repair Supports damaged nerves, relieves pain.	Basil, Peppermint, Helichrysum and Marjoram.	Apply to area of pain.
PMS Support Supports pre-menstrual discomforts	Vetiver, Clary Sage, Orange, Petitgrain, Sandalwood, Linden Blossom, Bergamot, Lemon Cinnamon and Neroli.	Apply across lower back, lower abdomen and around ankles
Purification Helps neutralize mold, mildew, fungus, airborne bacteria and viruses	Lemongrass, Rosemary, Tea Tree, Lavender, Myrtle and Citronella.	Diffuse or apply to infected areas.
Sinus Support Helps to clear and open the nasal passages and support the relief of sinus pressure from chronic sinus infections and/or sinus issues related to allergies	Thyme, Eucalyptus, Peppermint, and Lavender.	Apply 2 – 3 drops to a Q-tip and swabbing the inside of the nasal passages 2 – 6 times daily.
Sleep Supports restful sleep.	Orange, Tangerine, Patchouli, Blue Tansy, Lime, Spikenard, Ylang Ylang, Lavender, Chamomile and Citronella.	Apply to nape of the neck or bottom of feet.

To learn more about specific oils included in each blend and how they work to support specific organs and regions of the brain, visit https://vibrantblueoils.com/bookbonus/

About the Author

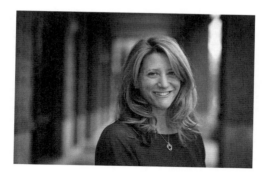

Jodi Sternoff Cohen is an award-winning journalist who has combined her training in nutritional therapy and aromatherapy to create unique proprietary blends of organic and wildcrafted essential oils that helped her heal her own anxiety, insomnia, and autoimmunity.

Recognizing that essential oils open a backdoor into the body through the olfactory system and topical application, she founded Vibrant Blue Oils (VibrantBlueOils.com) to empower practitioners and individuals with the knowledge and tools to heal the underlying imbalances that often lead to disease, including sleep, stress, digestion, systemic inflammation, detoxification, and blood-sugar dysregulation.

Her passion as researcher, clinician, educator, and mother drove her to share her story and her unique knowledge and experience in this book. She hopes to educate everyone interested in holistic wellness on the potential of essential oils to help the body heal.

In addition to her experience in natural healing, Jodi worked as a marketing executive at Microsoft, Time Inc., and US News & World Report. She holds an MBA from Columbia University and lives in Seattle, Washington, with her two children and her dog, Riley.

References

Chapter 1: Why Essential Oils Work

Terry Wahls, M.D., *The Wahls Protocol: A Radical New Way to Treat All Chronic Autoimmune Condtions Using Paleo Principles* (Penguin Group LLC: New York, New York, 2014)

Prof. (Dr.) Ciddi Veeresham, "Natural products derived from plants as a source of drugs." Journal of Advanced Pharmaceutical Technology & Research, Oct-Dec 2012 http://www.ncbi.nlm.nih.gov/pmc/articles/PMC3560124/

B.C. Freeman and G.A. Beattie. 2008. "An Overview of Plant Defenses against Pathogens and Herbivores". The Plant Health Instructor. DOI: 10.1094/PHI-I-2008-0226-01 2008 http://www.apsnet.org/edcenter/intropp/topics/Pages/OverviewOfPlantDiseases.aspx

Tori Rodriguez "Essential Oils Might Be the New Antibiotics" The Atlantic, Jan 16, 2015 http://www.theatlantic.com/health/archive/2015/01/the-new-antibiotics-might-be-essential-oils/384247/

Zava DT1, Dollbaum CM, Blen M. "Estrogen and progestin bioactivity of foods, herbs, and spices" Proceedings of the Society of Experimental Biology and Medicine, March 1998 http://www.ncbi.nlm.nih.gov/pubmed/9492350

Susanne Fischer-Rizzi, *Complete Aromatherapy Handbook: Essential Oils for Radiant Health* (Sterling Publishing Co., Inc.: New York, New York, 1990)

Clinton Ober, Stephen T. Sinatra, M.D. and Martin Zucker *Earthing: The Most Important Health Discovery Ever?* (Basic Health Publications, Inc.: Laguna Beach, California, 2010)

Valerie Ann Worwood, *Aromatherapy for the Soul: Healing the Spirit with Fragrance and Essential Oils* (New World Library: Novato, California, 1999)

Anthony William, *Medical Medium: Secrets Behind Chronic and Mystery Illness and How to Finally Heal* (Hay House, Inc.: Carlsbad, California, 2015)

Gotz Blome, M.D., *Advanced Bach Flower Therapy: A Scientific Approach to Diagnosis and Treatment* (Healing Arts Press: Rochester, Vermont, 1992)

Horst Rechelbacher, *Aveda Rituals: A Daily Guide to Natural Beauty and Health* (Henry Holt and Company, New York, 1999)

Masaru Emoto, *The Hidden Messages in Water* (Atria Books: New York and London, 2001)

Rev. Franklin Loehr, *The Power of Prayer on Plants* (Signet Books: New York, New York, 1959)

David Stewart Ph.D., D.N.M., *The Chemistry of Essential Oils Made Simple: God's Love Manifest in Molecules* Sixth Edition (Care Publications: Marble Hill, Missouri, 2016)

Chapter 2: How to Use Essential Oils

Robert Tisserand, Therapeutic Foundations of Essential Oils, http://tisserandinstitute.org, 2015

Jerry Tennant, MD, MD(H), MD(P), *Healing is Voltage: The Handbook* Second Edition (Jerry Tennant, 2011)

Higley, Connie and Alan *Reference Guide for Essential Oils* (Abundant Health, 2016)

David Stewart Ph.D., D.N.M., *The Chemistry of Essential Oils Made Simple: God's Love Manifest in Molecules* Sixth Edition (Care Publications: Marble Hill, Missouri, 2016)

Rupert Sheldrake, *Morphic Resonance & The Presence of the Past: The Habits of Nature* (Park Street Press: Rochester, Vermont, 1988)

Hans Jenny, *Cymatics: A Study of Wave Phenomena & Vibration* (MACROmedia Publishing, Newmarket, NH, 2001)

Chapter 3: The Parasympathetic State

Robert M. Sapolsky. *Why Zebras Don't Get Ulcers: An Updated Guide To Stress, Stress Related Diseases, and Coping.* (Henry Holt and Company, New York, 1998)

Lawrence Wilson "SYMPATHETIC DOMINANCE" http://drlwilson. com/Articles/SYMPATHETIC%20DOMINANCE.htm, August 2016

Dr. Stephen Porges, *The Polyvagal Theory: Neurophysiological Foundations of Emotions, Attachment, Communication, and Self-regulation*, (W. W. Norton & Company, New York, 2011)

Mark Hyman, *The UltraMind Solution: Fix Your Broken Brain by Healing Your Body First* (Simon & Schuster Audio, New York, 2008)

Chapter 4: Sleep

Sarah Ballantyne Go to Bed https://www.thepaleomom.com/books/gotobed/, 2015

Chapter 6: Emotions

Lissa Rankin, M.D., *The Fear Cure: Cultivating Courage as Medicine for the Body, Mind, and Soul* (Hay House, Inc.: Carlsbad, California, 2015)

Joseph LeDoux, *The Emotional Brain: The Mysterious Underpinnings of Emotional Life* (Simon & Schuster Paperbacks: New York and London, 1996)

Prof. Rachel S. Herz, "Do scents affect people's moods or work performance?", Scientific American https://www.scientificamerican.com/article/do-scents-affect-peoples/

Dr. Bradley Nelson, *The Emotion Code: How to Release Your Trapped Emotions for Abundant Health, Love and Happiness* (Wellness Unmasked Publishing: Mesquite, Nevada, 2007)

Louise Hay, *The Power is Within You* (Hay House: Carlsbad, California, 1991)

Lise Bourbeau *Your Body's Telling You: Love Yourself! The Most Complete Book on Metaphysical Causes of Illness and Disease* (Les Editions E.T.C. Inc.: Saint-Jerome (Quebec) Canada, 2001)

Chapter 8: Gut Repair and Inflammation

Sarah Ballantyne, *The Paleo Approach: Reverse Autoimmune Disease and Heal Your Body* (Victory Belt Publishing, Las Vegas, 2013). p. 302- 303.

Dr. Natasha Campbell-McBride, *Gut and Psychology Syndrome* (Medinform Publishing, Wymondham, Norfolk, United Kingdom, 2010)

Chapter 10: Brain Support: Blood Sugar and Circulation

Datis Kharrazian, *Why Isn't My Brain Working?: A Revolutionary Understanding of Brain Decline and Effective Strategies to Recover Your Brain's Health* (Elephant Press; Carlsbad, CA, 2013)

Other helpful resources

Jimm Harrison *Aromatherapy: Theraeutic Use of Essential Oils for Esthetics* (Milady - Cengage Learning: Clifton Park, New York, 2008)

Kurt Schnaubelt, Ph.D., *Advanced Aromatherapy: The Science of Essential Oil Therapy* (Healing Arts Press: Rochester, Vermont, 1998)

Kurt Schnaubelt, *Medical Aromatherapy: Healing with Essential Oils* (Frog Books: Berkeley, California, 1999)

Valerie Ann Worwood, *The Complete Book of Essential Oils and Aromatherapy: Over 800 Natural, Nontoxic, and Fragrant Recipes to Create Health, Beauty, and Safe Home and Work Environments* (New World Library: Novato, California, 2016)
Shirley Price, *Aromatherapy for Common Ailments: How to use Essential Oils— Such as Rosemary, Chamomile, and Lavender—to Prevent and Treat More than 40 Common Ailments* (Simon & Shuster: New York and London, 1991)

Susan Stockton *The Terrain is Everything: Contextual Factors That Influence Our Health* (Power of One Publishing: Clearwater, Florida, 2000)

Barbara Ann Brennan, *Hands of Light: A Guide to Healing Through the Human Energy Field* (Bantam Books: New York, New York, 1987)

Cyndi Dale, *The Subtle Body: An Encyclopedia of Your Energetic* (Sounds True: Boulder, Colorado, 2009)

Dr. LeAnne Deardeuff, DC and Dr. David Dearduff, DC *Inner Transformations Using Essential Oils: Powerful Cleansing Protocols for Increased Energy and Better Health* (Life Science Publishing: Orem, Utah, 2006)

Gabriel Mojay, *Aromatherapy for Healing the Spirit: Restoring Emotional and Mental Balance with Essential Oils* (Healing Arts Press: Rochester, Vermont, 1997)

Index